Advance Praise for *Triage*

"One of the joys of studying history is that people emerge from the shadows, whose actions that would otherwise have been forgotten, and demand our attention. The experiences of frontline medics revealed in full by the energetic researches of Martin King, who has demonstrated that they should be counted as history's true heroes."

—Peter Snow, historian, author,
and host of *20ᵗʰ Century Battlefields*

"Martin's stories reminds me of that which the soldiers in the 327ᵗʰ Infantry Brigade, 101ˢᵗ Airborne Division hold dear: selflessness, duty, and commitment. Medics are a shining example of these attributes and these stories reminds all of us in uniform that we must never forget the sacrifice and service of those who came before us. This is a must-read for anyone, and also those who have served, as well as their loving, supportive families."

—Colonel Rob Campbell (Retired),
Commander, 327ᵗʰ Infantry Regiment, 1ˢᵗ Brigade
Combat Team, 101ˢᵗ Airborne Division (Air Assault)

"Thanks to the passion and determination of Martin King to deliver the extraordinary details of these modern-day saints. Frontline medics do the right thing even in the face of hell!"

—Helen Patton, granddaughter
of General George Patton

This volume is dedicated to my dear friends Randy and Staci Garcia and the wonderful staff at ICC.

TRIAGE

A History of America's Frontline Medics
from Concord to Covid-19

MARTIN KING & MICHAEL COLLINS

A KNOX PRESS BOOK
An Imprint of Permuted Press
ISBN: 978-1-64293-976-7
ISBN (eBook): 978-1-64293-977-4

Triage:
A History of America's Frontline Medics from Concord to Covid-19
© 2021 by Martin King and Michael Collins
All Rights Reserved

Cover art by Cody Corcoran
Back cover photo by Nurse Allycia King

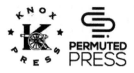

Permuted Press, LLC
New York • Nashville
permutedpress.com

Published in the United States of America
1 2 3 4 5 6 7 8 9 10

CONTENTS

FOREWORD BY BRIGADIER GENERAL (RET), ROBERT G. NOVOTNY, USAF

In my thirty years of flying combat fighter aircrafts, with five deployments to the Middle East and Afghanistan, I can tell you from personal experience that there are few treatments for the apprehension that fills your soul prior to war. Three things come to mind that can act as a mild remedy: First, the effectiveness and recency of your unit's training for combat. Second, the camaraderie and cohesiveness of the warfighting team. And finally, the knowledge that if you are wounded in war, there stands ready an amazing team of military combat physicians who will care for you, return you to your unit, or send you home to your family alive. 2021 marks the twentieth straight year of sustained combat operations in Afghanistan, and it is widely held that a revolution in military medicine has gone almost undetected. Credit to these military medics is well overdue, and the low numbers of combat casualties are but one metric to grade their success. While deployed, we spoke to military medical planning with the terms "Platinum 15" and the "Golden Hour." It was indisputable that if a military medic could attend to a wounded service member within fifteen minutes of initial injury, the likelihood of survival rocketed close to 95 percent. Furthermore, if that wounded service member was evacuated from the battlefield and transported to a combat medical facility within the first "Golden Hour," the results were even more noteworthy. This is a story worth telling and Martin King does exactly that in his newest historical work *Triage*. I met Martin in early 2019 when we both spoke at a military historical event in Las Vegas…a mere week or less before the United States began to restrict activities in response to the growing COVID-19 pandemic. His timely novel documenting the heroic work of military medics spans from the early American experiences in the pre-industrial age of warfare to the frontline caregivers fighting the pandemic in our very midst. Martin is a keen studier of war and an incredible storyteller, especially those stories that have had profound impacts on the lives of others. *Triage* is the story of those heroes.

Robert G. Novotny, Brig Gen (ret), USAF

INTRODUCTION

Just out of interest, "triage" is the medical process of determining the priority of patients' treatments by the severity of their condition, or likelihood of recovery with and without treatment. In other words, a person with suitable medical qualifications walks among the afflicted and determines whether or not someone should or shouldn't buy green bananas. The problem was that in the past the person charged with this great responsibility wasn't, as we will discover, always the right person for the job.

This volume begins and ends in the New World. While at the time of writing millions remain at home to minimize transmission of a severe acute respiratory syndrome aka COVID-19, across the states and around the world healthcare workers prepare to do the precisely the opposite. Social distancing demurs physical contact, but these remarkable individuals will put themselves in harm's way in the clinics, hospitals, and care homes or wherever they are sent. Numerous reports from medical staff describing the torment of difficult triage decisions and the anguish of losing patients and colleagues amount to a lexicon of physical and mental torment almost equivalent to a battlefield experience. They might not have to brave bullets and shrapnel, but they are confronted daily with the additional risk of infection. These angels carry on undeterred. This volume is a tribute to them, to the front line teams that have been saving lives since the American Revolutionary War. So while the world is being ravaged by this pandemic, what better excuse does one need to stay home and read a book?

The story begins in the days when the status of some women was gradually evolving from that of domestic pet and potential witch to essential caregiver on the battlefront. In the 18th century surgeons and nurses became an imperative rather than an additional luxury to armies in the field, where their intrinsic value far exceeded the paltry remuneration they received for their efforts to keep soldiers breathing. So not much has changed there. The nurses worked tirelessly alongside surgeons to patch up the wounded and either send them home, get them back on the front lines, or measure them up for a wooden overcoat. Not much has changed there either. Despite having little more than common sense and good housekeeping skills, these first impromptu nurses often had to serve under the auspices of grossly incompetent physicians (but men were always right back then, weren't they?).

It's almost a paradox that in the beginning, America's front line medical staff was comprised mostly of civilians, assisted by the military. Now, over three hundred years later, that appears to be the case again. Only this time no one can see the enemy, but they can see the terrible damage it can inflict on the victims. They can see the stricken faces of bereaved relatives who don't even have the luxury of sharing those last vital hours on earth with their loved ones in proximity. Relatives are forbidden from holding a hand or tenderly cradling the head of someone struggling to breathe their last breath, but the doctors and nurses aren't confined by such restrictions.

Front line medical teams are consummate experts at internalizing their grief, it goes with the turf, and this has always been the case. The fact that military medics are at higher risk of burnout, compassion fatigue, combat stress, and medic PTSD than their fellow combat personnel also applies to civilian health workers. They absorb the anguish and pain close relatives of the victims can't see, and they share their sadness and carry on regardless, repeating the same heart-rending processes day in day out.

Nevertheless, a war is a war, and an enemy remains an enemy until it is neutralized or completely eradicated.

Front line teams are stepping up to the plate as they have done on innumerable occasions in the past and will do again when called upon. The opening page of the US Department of Defense website reads, "The Defense Department is working closely with the Department of Health and Human Services and the State Department to provide support in dealing with the coronavirus."[1] Civilian and military authorities are working together again just like they did a very long time ago.

From the first American military engagements at Lexington and Concord to the hills and mountains of Afghanistan, then on to the fight against COVID-19, America's front line medical teams have braved arrows, bombs, bullets, and potentially fatal diseases to do their job. They have always gone the extra mile to be there for others, and if need be, to sacrifice their own lives to save others.

Back in 1775 Continental Army commanders came to realize the potential benefits of caring for (and even healing) the casualties of war. They realized a basic truth that had been long accepted as standard practice in European armies. It was better to patch a soldier up and get him back fighting than to administer a coup de grace and finish the poor fellow off.

These days a Red Cross or Red Crescent on armbands or helmets usually distinguishes front line medical personnel from other military belligerents, but this wasn't always the case. Through the ages the men and women who responded to the cry of "Medic!" were a remarkable collective indeed, unimpeded by race or ethnicity, and equally undefined by nationality or gender. They proved on innumerable occasions that care has no color and courage has no creed. The fight against COVID-19 is no exception. It is a war that still entails courageous, selfless individuals stepping up to the plate and risking their own lives to save others against this heartless, indiscriminate enemy. This volume is a small tribute to some truly exceptional human beings. Front line nurses, healthcare workers and medical staff in general epitomize what is best about the human

---

[1] "Homepage," U.S. Department of Defense (U.S. Department of Defense), accessed 4AD, https://dod.defense.gov/.

condition. This is what makes them exceptional. This is what makes them praiseworthy.

Back through the annals of military history, all serious military operations demanded trained medical staff. Pharaoh Ramses knew it and so did Emperor Julius Caesar, Napoleon, General Patton, along with many others—but it took time. It took a long time for the notion to hit home. Once the de facto rule was established, those encumbered by intransigent ideologies began to reassess the vital importance and the invaluable service trained medical personnel could provide. This development lead to the establishment of real front line medical services, but it was a tortuously painful road. As the volume progresses you will be able to read firsthand accounts from veterans of various wars and conflicts.

PREFACE

Despite being a terrible patient when the occasion has prevailed, I (author Martin King) dearly love, respect, and venerate all nurses and medics. I've written ten books on the subject of military history, but this is the one that hits home with me personally because I have been around people in the medical profession for most of my life. My mother was a nurse, my wife is a front line nurse and so is my daughter, one of my sisters, and my niece. My younger sister is also potentially exposed to danger working with crack and meth heads that have in some cases contracted COVID-19. Front line medical teams are, for me, among the finest and most resilient people I have ever known. I should also point out that they are drastically underpaid for the work they do. Quite a few of the nurses' smoke like brick factory chimneys, and they can all handle their drinks. What I find particularly amazing is their capacity to occasionally introduce levity into the proceedings. I love their acerbic, often black humor. So what if a few of them do prescribed meds? They're all still angels to me.

While I was deeply embroiled in the process of researching the story of a bi-racial nurse named Augusta Chiwy, who voluntarily committed herself to saving American lives in WWII, I began to nurture a fresh appreciation for the history of battlefield medicine and how it has evolved through the centuries. It was my dear friend Augusta who inspired me to look deeper into the subject.

Today medical teams around the world are fighting an unseen enemy in a global pandemic. The only good thing about COVID-19 is that it is indiscriminate and, as one American medic once said, mortality "is a great leveler." Mike Collins and I hope that this volume will inspire and entertain as we take you back through the ages and look at how the lives of those whose capacity for selfless dedication, intrepid innovation and ultimately human compassion managed to change the world. We hope that you will enjoy *Triage* as much as I enjoyed writing it.

PART 1

STARTING OUT

CHAPTER ONE

America's First Front Line Medics

Medical practice in America during the Pilgrim era was at best an exercise in "what will happen if I do this?" At worst it was potentially life threatening. To the Pilgrim Fathers that subscribed to archaic theories such as Hippocrates' "humors," treatment was based on herbalism, phlebotomy (the process of making a puncture in a vein for bloodletting from the patient's arm), fervent prayer and various herbal concoctions. Sickness and disease was a constant threat to these religious separatists, who had risked everything to secure religious freedom for themselves and their families. Apart from the actual Pilgrim Fathers, the Mayflower brought two relatively important medical resources to the New World. Deacon Samuel Fuller, who possessed some rudimentary medical knowledge and a copy of the book *The Surgeon's Mate* by Dr. John Woodall.[2] All medical practice in America during the Pilgrim era was an exercise in pure pragmatism. The author, Dr. John Woodall (1570–1643) began as a lowly barber-surgeon and rose to the position of first Surgeon General

---

2   Sir D'arcy Power, "V. The Surgeons Mate by John Woodall," BJS Society (John Wiley & Sons, Ltd, December 6, 2005), https://bjssjournals.onlinelibrary.wiley.com/doi/abs/10.1002/bjs.1800166102.

of England. He made a fortune stocking surgical chests and practiced at the Great St. Bartholomew Hospital in London for many years. The only other viable source of medical information would have been derived from the few Native Americans who lived in proximity to the settlers.

When the indigenous peoples of the Americas encountered European settlers for the first time in the 15th century, they were confronted with new religions, new customs, and tragically, new diseases. Plymouth Colony also had fewer Native Americans than expected because three years before the arrival of the Mayflower a decimating contagion had wiped out many coastal tribes, and within decades of those primary meetings a significant number of coastal indigenous populations had decreased almost to the point of extinction. Researchers have discovered that these diseases also reflect on modern-day populations of Native Americans. A recent study suggests that infectious diseases introduced by Europeans, such as smallpox and measles all those hundreds of years ago, have molded the immune systems of today's indigenous Americans.

It all started so well. The Native American Wampanoag tribe that resided in the area when the Pilgrim Fathers arrived, demonstrated to the Pilgrims how to smoke and dry indigenous fauna and fish, and how to plant corn, beans, and squash in mounds fertilized by fish and blessed by powdered tobacco, which incidentally is a very effective organic insect repellent. Shame that some idiot somewhere down the line said, "Have you tried smoking this?" Those first settlers also procured a plethora of invaluable information and knowledge from Native Americans on how to identify toxic plants, herbs, roots, barks, and berries along with the medicinal and culinary use of indigenous herbs and spices, and other naturally occurring biological components.

Precisely how or when Deacon Samuel became the physician for the New Plymouth colony isn't overtly apparent, but indications are that it all transpired as early as that first relatively mild winter of 1621. The way medicine was practiced in the 17th century bore little resemblance to the contemporary approach. For a start, medical practitioners hadn't always benefited from a formal education. It's entirely possible that Samuel gained his medical knowledge from on-the-job training and firsthand experience, which isn't necessarily a bad learning ground. The Pilgrims were not bothered in the slightest that their main physician was making it up as he went along, they were just happy to have someone in New Plymouth, and subsequently, in Massachusetts Bay, that possessed any medical knowledge.

More than fifty years before the Pilgrim Fathers landed the French physician Ambroise Paré, who appears again later in this volume, had published a book detailing his most effective surgical interventions. While the Pilgrim Fathers were taking steps to establish an effective colony in the New World, Europe was witnessing the emergence of the academic physician, where study of the medical arts was covetously divided between physician, surgeon, and apothecary. In the New World they needed all the help they could procure, and anyone practicing medicine needed to be all of these and then some. Just as the ancient Egyptians had done thousands of years previously, the Pilgrim Fathers regarded spiritual and corporeal matters as being inextricably linked. This explains why Samuel Fuller,[3] the first doctor in Massachusetts, was also a practicing deacon of the church.

This was in some respects a bad combination on many levels. Despite his numerous detractors, Samuel carried on undeterred because there was little or no alternative. He claimed that his experience had been gained from the two prominent seats of learning for medical education in London, England, and Leiden in the Netherlands, despite the fact that there's no evidence that Samuel ever benefited from a formal university education (in England, at least). There were some who regarded him as an unadulterated quack, but the patients wouldn't really have had the option of a second opinion. If all else failed there was always the big man upstairs to pray to, give thanks to, or blame, depending on the circumstances.

In the 16th and 17th centuries, western Europeans would call any fabric that had intimate contact with the body "linen." Rather than bathing with water and soap, Pilgrims, like their European relatives, trusted their cleanliness to a linen shirt or shift worn next to the skin beneath all

---

[3]   David R. Evans, "Samuel Fuller, Dr., the Pilgrim," Dr. Samuel Fuller, http://web.pdx.edu/~davide/gene/Fuller_Samuel_2.htm.

their other garments. The idea was that the linen was supposed to absorb all dirt and sweat from the body, rendering the cloth both an intimate and a potentially offensive item of clothing.[4] Unlike wealthy Europeans, Pilgrims could not afford to change or wash their shirts frequently, meaning that their dry baths were indeed seldom (hence on a dark night, one would smell them before one saw them).

For the early Americans at Plymouth, the concept of cleanliness incorporated the virtues of moral and spiritual purity, which were just as important as physical purity. Approximately 50 percent of the Mayflower survivors died in the first two months of 1621. William Bradford,[5] that staunch English Puritan separatist originally from the West Riding of Yorkshire in Northern England, attempted to establish a system of communal labor to encourage the efficiency of the survivors. This implied that women would even be required to launder the clothes of stinky men who were not even their husbands. There were some notably vociferous objections, but they fell on deaf ears at the time.

European ways and medical practices continued to have a direct influence on Continental ways and means right up until the advent of the Revolutionary Wars. When Congress appointed George Washington to command the Continental Army besieging Boston, they also selected Dr. Benjamin Church to be the first Director General and Chief Physician of the Hospital of the Army. At the onset of the Revolutionary War, male soldiers traditionally conducted nursing in the military; however, shortly after it began in 1775, a request was made by General Horatio Gates for a woman to care for his wounded soldiers. He informed the commander, "The sick suffer much for want of good female nurses." General George Washington officially asked Congress to provide female nurses to attend the sick and matrons to supervise the nurses.

In the 18th century, women were a visible part of any part of army encampment. Some of these women were the wives of soldiers who

[4] Greg Cook, "Did Pilgrims Bathe?—Asking About The First Thanksgiving At Plimoth Plantation," The ARTery (WBUR, November 14, 2014), https://www.wbur.org/artery/2014/11/14/thanksgiving-plimoth-plantation.

[5] History of Plymouth Plantation By William Bradford: Google Books.

simply trailed along, all dressed up and no place to go. Other women offered their services for pay as cooks, washerwomen, nurses, prostitutes, or seamstresses. Up until that time women were just regarded as wives, mothers, and sisters as well as caretakers of children, family, and community when they were in fact already nurses and care providers. The women endured the same hardships and deprivations that the soldiers endured and had been there.

The saying "an army marches on its stomach," attests to the importance of forces being well-provisioned. It has been attributed to both Napoleon and Frederick the Great. At Valley Forge during that punishing winter of 1777–1778 when Dr. Albigence Waldo,[6] a Continental Army surgeon, reported that many men survived largely on what were known as fire cakes (flour and water baked over coals). Waldo wrote that one retentive soldier complained that the reason for his retention was "my glutted guts are turned to pasteboard."[7]

Medical services provided by the Continental Army throughout most of the Revolutionary War were on the whole chronically disorganized and highly inefficient. There was a general lack of all provisions that was exacerbated by bitter infighting as the higher echelons jockeyed for precedence, power, and supplies that were provided for regiments and general hospitals. Poorly trained surgeons and the failure of general officers, including Washington, to appreciate the importance of the hospitals were the basic ingredients of disorder and failure.

It didn't help that the first three appointed Director Generals, who collectively directed the medical services from the summer of 1775 until January 1780, were all accused, in varying degrees, of incompetence and negligence. The first Surgeon General, who served as the Director General and Chief Physician of the Hospital of the Army from July 27, 1775, to October 17, 1775 was Dr. Benjamin Church. His popularity rating plummeted when he engaged in treasonable correspondence with

---

6   American Military History: A Documentary Reader. By Brad D. Lookingbill (John Wiley & Sons).

7   God Knows All Your Names: Stories in American History. By Paul N. Herbert (AuthorHouse).

the enemy and was promptly told to pick up his things on the way out. His successor Dr. John Morgan was held accountable for the terrible suffering and deprivation of the sick and wounded in the winter of 1776 and 1777. He got sacked, too. The third Director, Dr. William Shippen, Jr., had only just assumed the post when he became the subject of some vitriolic criticism, mainly from the two previous occupants of this office. The fervent squabbling and backbiting culminated with Shippen's court martial, and though acquitted and reappointed, he didn't stick around to watch the paint dry and quit the service in disgust. The final appointment during the Revolutionary Wars in the late winter of 1780–1781 was James Tilton of Delaware, who managed to appease most factions and restore some order to the supply and medical care services.

The often-vicious infighting between two of these notables, namely Dr. John Morgan and Dr. William Shippen, Jr., wasn't conducive to good governance. Wee Willy's dad, William Shippen, Sr. (1712–1801), had been a respected medical doctor in Philadelphia, one of the founders of the Pennsylvania Hospital in 1753, and a member of the Continental Congress elected in 1778. This probably set the stage for William Shippen, Jr. In January 1780, Shippen was arrested and accused of five specific charges. His accusers claimed that Shippen had speculated with supplies such as wine and sugar at a time when the sick and wounded were in desperate need, and further asserted that his incompetence caused needless suffering and death. Following a highly improper trial, during which the board's composition changed with alarming regularity and the accused privately entertained the board members with fine food and mocking imitations of his principal detractor Dr. John Morgan, Shippen escaped conviction by one vote. His steadfast defense of his conduct confirmed the general consensus of opinion that he was insensitive to human suffering. It's true that he never went out of his way to visit the sick, never dressed a wound or offered comfort to the soldiers. Despite this, Shippen remained in the position until his resignation on January 3, 1781. He survived the ensuing scandal and went on to have an illustrious career in the former colony.

Shippen contributed significantly to the establishment of medicine in America as a profession based on university training. He also pioneered courses in midwifery despite opposition from "the unskilled old women," whose methods he believed caused needless suffering and sometimes death. He provided scientific knowledge about women's diseases and appropriate treatments, along with "necessary cautions against the dangerous and cruel use of instruments." He died of anthrax on July 11, 1808, in Germantown, Philadelphia.

The life of one future president of the United States was saved at the Battle of Trenton when a musket ball pierced his shoulder and severed an artery. Fortunately there was a doctor on hand to patch him up and send him on his way. Monroe had been sent to keep an eye on a road that led out of Trenton. While assuming his post, he created enough noise to rattle the dogs that belonged to a local doctor who was not impressed. It was 0200 when the doctor approached Monroe to inquire after the source of this disturbance. Monroe explained the situation and Dr. John Riker offered to accompany him. This was a fortuitous alignment because Riker was on hand when Monroe caught the musket ball.[8]

The actions at Valley Forge exemplified and personified the deficiencies in the Continental Army's supply system, imperfect at best, and on occasion it completely imploded causing unimaginable misery. Everyone was freezing, starving, and some were probably feeling homesick because in the 18th century, home and hearth was the epicenter of everything, particularly health care. Even after the nation's first hospital opened in Philadelphia in 1751, another century would have to pass before the public would come to regard hospitals as reputable and safe, and even then there would be those who maintained certain reservations at the prospect of hospitalization.

Once it had been agreed that women were indeed well qualified and up to the task, the Continental army replaced most male nurses with preferred female nurses. To provide a means of caring for sick soldiers, Congress also authorized the formation of hospitals.

---

[8] The Presidents: Noted Historians Rank America's Best and Worst Chief Executives – The Presidents. By Brian Lamb, Susan Swain (Hachette).

In July 1775 a plan was devised to allocate one nurse to every ten patients and one matron for every one hundred wounded or sick soldiers. This was the first instance of some sort of organized nursing system in the military. Congress allowed a salary of two dollars per month for these nurses; matrons were paid four dollars per month. Nurses serving British soldiers received thirteen shillings per month. All female nurses were required to do mostly custodial work, feeding and bathing patients, emptying chamber pots, cleaning hospital wards, and occasionally cooking. They also changed linen, swept, disinfected hospitals with vinegar, combed hair, and were compelled to remain sober at all times. Nurses kept the hospitals and camps running. Despite Congressional efforts to increase the number of female nurses for the army, there remained a shortage throughout the war as Regiments constantly sought women to nurse their sick and wounded. The generals and officers of these regiments sometimes used nefarious means to coerce women into working as nurses, even threatening to withhold rations from women who refused to volunteer. The word "volunteer" probably had a different connotation in the military.

Revolutionary War nurses, military personnel, and medical professionals were constantly reliant on each other. It served as a good learning experience for future standards and procedures in military organization.

One of America's first front line medics was a gentleman by the name of Joseph Warren[9] who extolled his interest in matters medical shortly after enrolling at Harvard at the tender age of fourteen. By the age of twenty-two, he had qualified to become the youngest doctor in Boston. Among his patients he could flagrantly name-drop Samuel Adams, John Hancock, and future presidents John Adams and John Quincy Adams. Word travelled fast in the colonies in the 18th century, and Dr. Warren quickly built a solid reputation as one of Boston's finest physicians. This powerful position gave him access to prominent Loyalists, including the children of Royal Governor Thomas Hutchinson, British General

---

[9] Founding Martyr: The Life and Death of Dr. Joseph Warren, the American. By Christian Di Spigna (Crown).

Thomas Gage, and his rather naughty American-born wife, Margaret. Dr. Warren, it should be noted, was also an irrepressible philanderer.

Thanks to his medical practice and enthusiasm for illicit horizontal jogging, Dr. Warren could actively spy on the British. Being a young handsome doctor gave rise to rather juicy and not entirely unsubstantiated rumors that he was doing much more than applying soothing poultices to the afflicted parts. Some have even speculated that the widowed doctor may have carried on a fiery extramarital affair with Margaret Gage. This privileged position, missionary or otherwise, allowed Dr. Warren to obtain advanced notice of planned British troop movements to Concord on April 18, 1775.

Warren participated in the Lexington and Concord engagements as both a soldier and a doctor. He was selected to be the president of the Provincial Congress and the Rebellion's executive leader of the colony on May 31, 1775. He understood the importance of acquiring support for the American cause in Britain, so he convinced Congress to allow him to sail to England to deliver his account of the April battles to Benjamin Franklin in London. His letters reached England and were widely distributed by Franklin, causing quite a stir, and in some cases extreme embarrassment to polite society, the British government and the King (who hadn't exhibited any outward signs of his impending madness at the time, but would eventually hear voices and discuss weighty matters of state with flower beds and privet hedges). Dr. Warren told Franklin to disseminate his vital information to all British citizens that the Americans would sell their liberty "only at the price of their own lives."[10] Franklin was only too happy to acquiesce.

On June 14, 1775, Congress bestowed the rank of major general on Warren. In 1761 he had been inducted into one of the two Masonic lodges that were present in Boston at the time. He had chosen to join the newly established St. Andrew's lodge even though the other lodge, St. John's, was fiscally more promising and had more conservative and wealthy members. The reason he went for St. Andrew's was because

---

[10] Proceedings, Volume 22 Front Cover Baylor Research Foundation, 2009.

among its members were revolutionaries such as John Hancock and Paul Revere. Dr. Warren claimed to have had a confidential informer who had connections to the higher echelons of the British command. He never revealed the identity of the informant, but it wasn't such an intriguing mystery. Most historians have dismissed the Mrs. Gage connection as pure conjecture and some claim Warren may even have seen the British soldiers mustering for himself. He lived in relatively close proximity to the Green where the British Army was assembling. It is also entirely possible that Warren knew quite quickly after the boats mustered and the embarkation began, so he could give Revere the message to light two lanterns in the Old North Church, "two if by sea."[11] Before Warren dispatched an alarm rider, he would have ascertained that firm proof had been established, preferably firsthand proof.

So, shortly before those first military engagements, Dr. Warren dispatched Paul Revere and William Dawes on their famous "Midnight Ride" to warn the militia at Lexington and Concord and spread the alarm that the British were setting out to raid the town of Concord and arrest rebel leaders John Hancock and Samuel Adams. The dynamic duo Revere and Dawes arrived in Lexington within half an hour of each other. Then they set off again on their weary steeds to warn the residents of Concord of the impending British arrival. This time Dr. Samuel Prescott joined them. Prescott had ridden, during the evening of April 18, 1775, to call on his intended Lydia Mulliken, the daughter of a Lexington clockmaker who probably appreciated punctuality. On the way home, early in the morning of April 19, he learned that Paul Revere and William Dawes had brought the news that the British were on the march from Boston. Although the information they wanted to relay wasn't entirely correct it would give local the militia sufficient time to move military supplies out of Concord and conceal them in surrounding communities.

The problem was that before they could reach Concord, the three riders ran into a British patrol around 1:30 a.m. and Revere was captured. Prescott and his horse navigated a stone wall and managed to reach

---

11 Manual of Forensic Odontology, Fifth Edition. Edited by David R. Senn, Richard A. Weems CRC

Concord. One story claims that Dawes outwitted two British officers that were tailing him. Noticing that his horse was exhausted, he rode up to a farmhouse and allegedly shouted as if there were patriots residing at the property, "Hello boys, I've got me two of 'em!"[12] Fearing an imminent ambush, the two Redcoats turned tail and galloped away while Dawes' horse reared up so abruptly, he was physically ejected from the saddle. Prescott arrived at Concord around 1:30 a.m. to initiate a chain of alarms beginning with Colonel Barrett and the Concord militia. Afterward he rode to Acton and then possibly to Stow. While in Concord he triggered the alarm to his brother Abel Prescott who rode to Sudbury and then Framingham. By the time the British reached Lexington they could hear alarms going off and horses galloping. The secret British march quickly became public knowledge to the men of Massachusetts, and while Paul Revere became one of the darlings of the revolution, William Dawes and Dr. Prescott rode off into obscurity and were rarely heard from again.

During the ensuing battles of Lexington and Concord, Dr. Warren was courageous to the point of being reckless. It wasn't unusual for Continental doctors to do considerably more than tend the wounded. While tending the aforementioned, he frequently exposed himself to vigilant British sharp shooters who released a few musket balls in his direction, one of which glanced against a pin from his ear-lock musket and could have inflicted serious damage. This ominous precursor of things to come meant he survived the Battles of Lexington and Concord and lived to fight another day. Another doctor, Dr. Downer of Roxbury, actually engaged in single combat with a British soldier, who he expertly dispatched with a single well-aimed bayonet thrust. Being a doctor, Roxbury knew precisely how to angle the thrust to exact maximum damage, which was a bit of a "downer" for the Brit. There is no evidence that nurses were employed to tend the wounded at Concord or Lexington, but steps had been taken to provide nurses for future engagements.

Warren's bravery and loyalty were rewarded when, shortly before June 17, he was commissioned as a Major General in the colony's militia. Sadly,

---

[12] THE HISTORIE BOOKE A TALE OF TWO WORLDS AND FIVE CENTURIES. By The Ancient and Honorable Artillery Company (1903).

he wouldn't survive to receive the actual commission. On that date he voluntarily offered to join the assembled militia defending Breed's Hill (often mistakenly described as the Battle of Bunker Hill). By the time he arrived on the hill that overlooked Boston, Colonel William Prescott had lost many men during the night. Most of them had retired to the rear, and some had no immediate plans to return. The remaining front line soldiers were tired and haggard after a long night's digging and were foraging for supplies in the hope of receiving reinforcements. Meanwhile the British had landed and were forming ranks in preparation for the attack. Warren met Putnam beside a rail fence. David Putnam records the following conversation in his 1818 publication. After Putnam offered command to Warren, Warren replied, "I am here only as a volunteer. I know nothing of your dispositions; nor will I interfere with them. Tell me where I can be most useful." Putnam directed him to Prescott's redoubt on Breed's Hill.

As the final British assault began to breach the walls of the redoubt, Warren remained with the covering force. After the battle, there was some confusion concerning his fate. Some assumed that he had survived the battle while others couldn't agree on exactly how he had died. The details of the events on Breed's Hill remained veiled until the following year when Paul Revere helped identify Warren's body by using what might have been America's first case of forensic dentistry. Revere recognized Warren's false teeth that had been implanted years earlier.

Warren's remains indicated that cause of death was due to a musket ball that had struck his head. Closer analysis of the skull helped to reveal the truth about what occurred at Breed's Hill on that fateful day. He was not shot while retreating with the rest of the soldiers because the smaller bullet wound in Warrens' left maxilla and the larger exit wound in the right occiput illustrates that the bullet's trajectory crossed the midline of the brain, which most likely injured the brainstem. This proved unequivocally that he was facing the British, which corresponds with the most popular account that claims the very last militiamen had left the redoubt with great haste before a musket ball impacted Warrens' head and the poor man was killed outright.

As the weeks passed it became blatantly obvious that the army preferred female nurses to male, not only because they considered women better at caring for the sick but also because every woman nursing meant one more man was available to fight on the battlefield; however, women were not always eager to volunteer for nursing duty. Washington claimed that this was due to a fiscal consideration, and blamed the low compensation rate for the shortage of nurses. In 1776, Congress increased nurses' pay to four dollars a month,[13] and a year later it doubled again to eight dollars a month. It still didn't get anywhere near the princely sum of forty dollars per month that surgeons and apothecaries used to get paid. Some things never change. Thankfully they didn't have to contend with cosmetic surgeons.

Despite ongoing Congressional efforts to increase the number of women nurses for the army, throughout the war there were never really enough at any given time. Regiments constantly sought women to nurse their sick and wounded. In the spring of 1776 the General Hospital in Massachusetts desperately needed nurses for Cambridge and Roxbury, but there were many reasons why the profession of nursing wasn't initially attractive to ladies of the day. Serving as a nurse in the Continental Army was a precarious choice of vocation for a start. Although the women received regular pay and job security was relatively good, nursing in the army was potentially life-threatening. Today nurses are still exposed to deadly diseases, such as COVID-19 and Ebola. Back in 1775 they had to contend with smallpox, typhus, and cholera, any of which could cause premature death. Polite society refused to regard nursing as a respectable profession for ladies, and it was definitely not a métier for the fainthearted. Well-bred ladies of the late 18th century often struggled to maintain consciousness when faced with even the slightest emotional or physical shock, and nursing would have been a shock to the system for the less resilient back then as it still is today.

Throughout the American Revolutionary War, diseases (rather than battle injuries) were the main causes of death among the ranks, and

---

[13] "First Women Nurses," History of American Women, January 29, 2021, https://www.womenhistoryblog.com/2014/07/first-women-nurses.html.

nurses were often compelled to do the filthiest jobs associated with the medical profession. Officers would often have the temerity to threaten and withhold rations from women who refused to volunteer to work as nurses. These officers were known as total bastards, among other things, because precisely how valuable nurses were to Washington's army is borne out by the story of one remarkable Philadelphia housewife, nurse, and ad hoc spy named Lydia Darragh.[14]

According to legend on the night of December 2, 1777, Lydia single-handedly saved the lives of General George Washington and his whole Continental Army when she overheard the British planning a surprise attack on Washington's army scheduled for the following day. Previous pages have already testified to the incompetence of the British planning anything regarded as "secret." Whether there was an actual surprise attack planned or whether the story was simply contrived and disseminated to elevate the status of nurses has never been definitively ascertained, but at that time nurses needed all the good PR they could get. Lydia Darragh became another folk hero.

When contemporary historians and students are asked about the American Revolutionary War, they are probably more inclined to cite the names of George Washington, Benjamin Franklin, or Paul Revere, but probably not Molly Pitcher, Lydia Darragh, or Deborah Sampson. Granted the fiercely patriotic Deborah Sampson didn't work strictly as a nurse, but she had some ability in that department, and may even have been one of America's first cross-dressers. In 1782 she disguised herself as a man, unofficially changed her name to Robert Shurtleff, and joined the 4th Massachusetts Regiment (also known as the 3rd Continental Regiment or Learned's Regiment) where she served with great distinction as a soldier.

At West Point she was assigned to Captain George Webb's Company of Light Infantry. Some time later Deborah displayed incredible tenacity and dexterity when she physically extracted a musket ball from her own thigh, but it wasn't until she was actually knocked unconscious and sent

---

[14] Lydia Darragh, of the Revolution. By Henry Darrach, David Bacon, John Drinker and Geo. J. Scattergood (University of Pennsylvania Press).

to the hospital that surgeons noticed something missing in the lower groin area. She later recovered completely and was granted an honorable discharge and a military pension from the state of Massachusetts. In 1802 she became the first woman in America to organize a year-long lecture tour, relating her wartime experiences to enthralled audiences (there wasn't a lot of entertainment about), sometimes dressing in full military uniform just for effect. Four years after her death at age sixty-six, her toadying husband petitioned Congress for remuneration, seeing as he was the spouse of a former soldier. Although the couple was not actually married at the time of her service, in 1837 the committee concluded that the history of the Revolution "furnished no other similar example of female heroism, fidelity and courage." He was awarded the money, but in a sore twist of fate this freeloader died before receiving it.

Lydia Darragh was a feisty Irish woman born in Dublin, Ireland (1729–1789), and a confirmed Quaker who lived with her husband William and her family in Pennsylvania. During the war and due to the family's religious persuasion, the British erroneously assumed that all Quakers were pacifists and this innocuous family would remain neutral in the war. Nothing could have been further from the truth. Lydia had a son serving in the 2nd Pennsylvania Regiment with General George Washington's Army. This was one of the reasons she was more than prepared to work as a spy as well as a nurse. The other reason was that she lived on Second Street in Philadelphia, directly opposite British army HQ in Pennsylvania. According to legend, during the night of December 2, 1777, nurse Lydia Darragh single-handedly saved the lives of General George Washington and his Continental Army when she overheard the British planning a surprise attack scheduled the following day. Using a bit of Irish blarney and a carefully concocted story that she needed to buy flour from a nearby mill in proximity to the British line, Lydia passed this vital information on to American Lieutenant Colonel Thomas Craig. The legend was born. Whether or not it is entirely true is debatable, but nurses at the time were particularly efficient when it came to multi-tasking, and didn't someone once say, "Never let the truth get in the way of a good story?"[15]

Molly Pitcher was another legendary figure feted during and since the American Revolutionary War. The only problem with her is, well, no one is actually 100 percent sure that she existed at all. The name was a nickname attributed to a woman who was said to have carried water to thirsty American soldiers during the Battle of Monmouth on June 28, 1778, before taking over for her husband on the battlefield after he was incapacitated. The bucket she carried was known as a pitcher and many women were called Molly, hence "Molly Pitcher" was usually a request.

Truth is there is no real tangible proof that Molly Pitcher ever existed, but some claim that she did and that her real name was Mary Hays McCauley. Born in Pennsylvania in 1754 (or possibly 1744), she may have worked as a servant before marrying William Hays, of Carlisle, Pennsylvania who served as a gunner in the 4th Artillery of the Continental Army during the war. This particular Molly was part of the group of women, camp followers, who traveled with the army and took on such duties as cooking, washing, nursing the sick, and tending wounded soldiers. Whether Molly Pitcher was real or not became superfluous because the legend and the good PR alone was powerful enough to endorse the cause of women nurses.

Military orders for the Pennsylvania battalions stationed at Ticonderoga in July of 1776 stated that one woman be chosen from each company to go to the hospital at Fort George to nurse the sick. Documents for the hospital at Albany in July 1777 record employing nine female nurses. In 1778, General Washington ordered his regimental commanders to employ as many nurses as possible to aid regimental surgeons, and in 1781 he wrote a letter to Benjamin Franklin's daughter Sarah who was the leader of an association of women who purchased dry goods with their own money and sewed shirts for soldiers. He wrote: "Amidst the distress and sufferings of the Army, whatever sources they have arisen, it must be a consolation to our Virtuous Country Women that they have

---

[15] A Little Book of Random Quotes. By Kurt Vogler (self-published).

never been accused of withholding their most zealous efforts to support the cause we are engaged in."[16]

The virtuous countrywomen who offered their services to the army were embarking on a journey that offered discomfort, hardship, and was fraught with danger. In addition to supporting the army and its irrefutable cause, they struggled to make a living for themselves and their families. The contributions of Revolutionary War era women may have long since been assigned to posterity, but it's equally important to recount their bravery and sacrifice in the same breath as the fighting men they supported.

According to the classified ads of July 1776 in the Virginia Gazette that was printed in Williamsburg, General Nathaniel Greene advertised a request for nurses. "The sick being numerous in the hospital and but few women nurses to be had, the regimental surgeon must report the number necessary for the sick of the regiment and the colonels are requested to supply accordingly."

General Washington had both surgeons and physicians in his ranks because in the 18th century the title "surgeon" or "physician" implied different statures. A continental surgeon was regarded as a skilled technician, but not accorded the professional title on the European continent. Those Europeans could be incredibly snotty without any provocation. Anyway, those who performed little or no surgery were simply referred to as physicians. All surgeons are physicians, but not all physicians are surgeons.

A surgeon probably had to possess the skill, speed, and aloofness of a "hit man" to conduct his work with success and efficiency. If only they had read hieroglyphics or stories of the Greek and Romans. Hippocrates, the renowned Greek physician of the Age of Pericles whose name is eponymous with the famous oath once said, "He who desires to practice surgery must go to war."[17] What he implied was that only during warfare could a physician or a surgeon truly learn his art—closing wounds, treating infection, and learning the intricacies of human anatomy in

---

[16] The Journal of American History, Volume 7; Volume 13. Edited by Francis Trevelyan Miller.

[17] Homer: The Iliad. William Allan.

the hope of becoming skilled at using the variety of surgical and other medical instruments. In times of peace, doctors had few opportunities of perfecting their trade.

It was battlefield experience that helped to provide a new direction to the medical profession of this fledgling nation. Consequently, the primary training ground for the surgery of trauma in the 18th century America was indeed war. It provided many physicians and surgeons plenty of raw materials to practice on, and consequently great advances were made. Excessive exposure to injury and disease was ultimately necessary to progress in the field of medicine. The aftermath of a battle is where knowledge could be acquired by practice and observation. The often-horrific injuries that were incurred during the battles gave physicians and surgeons the opportunity to see and experience more in one day than they could have experienced in years of a peace time medical practice.

During war, men could sustain a variety of horrendous wounds inflicted by low velocity weapons, and some had limbs removed swiftly by flying cannon balls that could tear a gaping blood-stained hole in two or three ranks of men. A soldier's wound could also come from a musket ball, bayonet, sword or an Indian arrow, or a tomahawk. Low-maintenance barbers, aka the scalp collectors, could also do terrible damage. A soldier could succumb to a variety of terrible injuries. Therefore, the nurses had to be just as resilient as the surgeons who removed the parts when it came to enduring the agonizing screams and recriminations of the unfortunate wounded men. Many of those women were mothers and no strangers to agonizing pain. Burns were particularly fearsome because there was no widely available analgesic to treat them with.

Treating a major burn injury in the 18th century was little different from that described by French surgeon André Paré[18] during the battle of Turin in 1536 when he saw three grievously burned soldiers lying in a stable. As Paré inspected the severity of the wounds, an old soldier who

---

[18] La Méthode de traicter les playes faictes par hacquebutes et aultres bastons à feu et de celles qui sont faictes par flèches, dardz et semblables, aussy des combustions spécialement faictes par la pouldre à canon, composée par Ambroyse Paré,... Paris: V. Gaulterot. fol. 52 v.13. By André Paré (1545).

asked if there was any way to cure them joined him. "I said no, and then he went up to them and cut their throats, gently and without ill will toward them. Seeing this great cruelty, I told him he was a villain. He answered that he 'prayed God when he should be in such a plight, he might find someone to do the same for him, that he should not linger in misery.'" The coup de grace was often used to treat more serious injuries, and there were rumors that some women in the hospital were not above putting a pillow over the face of a badly wounded man and dispatching his soul to the Lord. In the words of Abigail Adams who wrote a poignant letter to her husband John Adams on March 31, 1776, "I desire you would remember the ladies."[19]

---

[19] Familiar Letters of John Adams and His Wife Abigail Adams, During the American Revolution. By John Adams, Charles Francis Adams.

CHAPTER TWO

Washington's Doc in Action

By the time the Revolutionary War was underway the situation in the colonies hadn't really improved all that much. Physicians and surgeons had introduced some new ideas, but they were still lacking in practical applications.

The Continental Congress officially created the American Continental Army on June 14, 1775. The following day, George Washington was selected to lead the nascent forces that had congregated around Boston. July 3, 1775, was another momentous date in that same seminal year in the history of this war (1775–1783). Freshly appointed Washington arrived at Cambridge, Massachusetts, to assume command of a Continental Army of approximately twenty thousand men strong that he would eventually lead to glory. According to the small print this appointment included taking full responsibility for the care of hospitalized sick and wounded soldiers that were mainly from the Massachusetts area. This didn't appear to be all that problematic because up until that juncture, Massachusetts' regimental surgeons had treated the wounded at Massachusetts facilities. Then some bright spark said, "What if the fighting spreads?" It soon became glaringly obvious to all but the blissfully ignorant that if the fighting extended to other states, the existing arrangement would definitely not suffice.

In 1775 it wasn't even deemed necessary to have previous military experience to qualify as an army physician. Consequently, the practitioners were not always medically qualified. The soldiers knew the butchers from the bakers. They knew the difference between competent and negligent, and it wasn't unusual for the stricken soldier's comrades to frag or even dispose of the offending cutter. Recovery was strictly arbitrary, and not always based on established medical procedures. The surgeons were at best an ad hoc collective with dubious references; at worst they could be more dangerous than the enemy. The American Army's Medical Department formed in 1775 was comprised of civilian practitioners, many of whom were quite impervious to possessing any medical knowledge and demonstrably self-trained. This information would spread like wildfire among the troops and wouldn't necessarily inspire their confidence.

July 27, 1775, was another important date in the Revolutionary War calendar because the Continental Congress approved a minor resolution authorizing the creation of a functional Hospital Department to provide for this recently assembled Continental Army. The fact that surgeons and physicians expected to serve in the army would not be given any military rank initially caused some consternation, but that soon dissipated as more pressing concerns arose. For a start there was the drastic shortage of drugs and medicines. In response to the latter, in September 1775 the Continental Congress created a "Medical Committee" whose sole remit was "to devise ways and means to supplying the Continental Army with Medicines."[20] So the rule of thumb in 1775 was "when in doubt start a committee."

A few committees later, Continental Congress authorized and approved the allocation of one surgeon to serve in each regiment. Not many of the freshly appointed regimental surgeons had any actual "hands on" experience with triage or treating trauma, but this wasn't regarded as a deterrent. They were mostly the sons of the privileged, trained through

---

[20] The Medical Department of United States Army from 1775 to 1873. By United States Surgeon General's Office.

the apprenticeship system at one of the two medical schools in the United States. The first medical college to be opened in America was in Philadelphia (now known as Pennsylvania University), which offered medical training. While some surgeons were trained at the Pennsylvania Hospital, founded in 1751 by Dr. Thomas Bond and Benjamin Franklin, others attended Kings College (now Columbia University) in New York. Because these colleges accepted only a handful of students for training, most American physicians were trained through apprenticeships and expected to endure seven years on the job before they were officially considered qualified to work as physicians.

Inexperienced physicians were a constant detriment to the troops in the field, and were in some cases feared more than the enemy. In their defense, some of these quacks were great entertainers and knew how to hold a crowd.

One particularly incompetent physician used to recommend trephination for nigh on every malady. He claimed that drilling a golf-ball-sized hole in someone's skull was always efficacious, even if it was occasionally lethal.

The previous century had seen the advent of tentative steps taken to perfecting the art of performing cranial surgery, and by the 18th century most aspiring neurosurgeons even kept their fingernails long in the event that they needed to remove an exposed pericranium. A good manicure always added that extra bit of theatricality to the drilling process, which was guaranteed to pull a crowd and extract gasps of "ooh" and "aww" and "poor bastard" from the assembled throng who soaked up every minute—until it was their turn. When all else failed, a good al fresco trephination was actually one of the few camp activities, apart from gambling and whoring, which gave the camp followers a breather.

Thanks to predecessors such as André Paré and Andreas Vesalius, most of Washington's physicians possessed a rudimentary knowledge of anatomy; however, precisely how the brain functioned would remain a complete mystery for a few decennia. Anything inexplicable was always easy to deal with. It was either the work of God, the Devil, or those time-honored party poopers (the evil spirits who could always be counted on in the blame game). Superstition was rampant and some astrologer-surgeons even believed that it was dangerous to use a trephine (the actual instrument used to drill the offending hole to remove a circle of tissue or bone) during a full moon because they thought that on such occasions the brain was enlarged and too close to the patient's skull.[21]

There is, however, evidence to propose that some practitioners were aware of the phenomenon of a post-traumatic cerebral edema, even if they didn't entirely comprehend the underlying mechanism. One surgeon recommending trephination for a comminuted fracture of the skull stated, "This should be undertaken when the patient had recovered from the immediate shock but not after the third day, the operation would then be fraught with danger."

A skillfully executed trephination would always provide a bloodthirsty spectacle for the spectators who had seriously distorted views on precisely what constituted entertainment. It is, however, safe to assume that the recipient of the surgeon's attention rarely expressed gratitude or jocularity while undergoing the treatment because (like most operations back then) it was usually performed without any kind anesthetic. Opium and rum were available, but usually reserved for the officers. Privates were expected to "bite down on this piece of wood," so it is doubtful that the patient (or victim, depending on one's perspective) had much regard for the person holding the trephine drill or sharpening the saw to remove a damaged extraneous limb.

One eminent but ever-so-slightly deranged physician of the day wrote: Females are liable to many diseases, which do not afflict the other sex.[22] Besides, the nervous system being more irritable in them than in men, their diseases were required to be treated with greater caution. They are less able to bear large evacuations, and all stimulating medicines ought to be administered to them with a sparing hand. (Apparently the rather precarious evacuation known as childbirth didn't count.)

---

[21] The Collective Evidence of Trephination of the Human Skull in Great Britain During Prehistoric Times. By Wilson T. Parry.

[22] On the Diseases Peculiar to Females: A Treatise Illustrating Their Symptoms. By Thomas John Graham.

For example, a delicate person with weak nerves who lives mostly within doors must not be treated, under any disease, precisely in the same manner as one who is hardy, robust, and much exposed to the open air. Doesn't that inspire confidence? In other words, deep thinkers and weaklings need not apply to join. So the conclusion there is women get ratty, don't do large dumps, and those of a sensitive nature should get out more often.

The colonial physicians who formed the American Army's Medical Department in 1775 were all civilian practitioners. Many had no prior military experience, and only a small percentage had actually earned M.D. degrees. Most were either apprentice or self-trained, and not many of them made any attempt to specialize in the manner customary in Europe where a choice was usually made among medicine, surgery, and pharmacy. The allegiance of appointed regimental surgeons tended to orient toward the regiment they served rather than the respective Hospital Department, which was frequently rendered ineffective thanks to disruptive bureaucratic infighting.

During the Revolutionary War, immediate management and stabilization of potentially life-threatening injury or illness resulting from combat took a back seat. The emphasis appears to have been on treating contagious disease, which accounted for most of the mortality during the period. One of the main problems surgeons and physicians frequently encountered was caused by the lack of consensus regarding treatment in general. Unfettered by the claustrophobic parameters of European guild traditions, American medicine could set its own agenda. This was all well and good, but it often exacerbated the situation rather than solve it. Furthermore, the effort to develop and establish fundamental concepts reduced the importance of the diagnosis of specific diseases. If that wasn't bad enough, there wasn't even consensus on what to call a specific disease. Back in merry old England, it was believed that a touch from royalty could heal a very unpopular skin disease known as scrofula or the "King's evil."[23] Well that was going to be a bit of a problem in America for obvious

---

[23] A Treatise on Struma Or Scrofula, Commonly Called the King's Evil. By Thomas White. U.a. Murray (1784).

reasons. Scrofula was usually indicated by an unsightly swelling of the lymph nodes in the neck caused by tuberculosis.

Most treatments were fairly statutory and consisted mainly of administering leeches for the purposes of bleeding and purging, and hot steam for blistering (regardless of the symptoms). Since surgery alone was confined mostly to theory rather than any significant degree of experience, it was always a very hit and miss affair when one had to go under the knife. If a battle injury revealed compound fractures, many surgeons favored immediate amputation. The danger was that in a hospital environment, the patient was vulnerable to wounds becoming infected, making amputation an imperative rather than a choice. Some surgeons preferred to postpone amputation until there was absolutely no alternative because the process didn't always save the patient's life.

When a damaged leg was removed at mid-thigh, the mortality rate was often between 45 and 65 percent. Dr. John Jones believed that immediate amputation was definitely advisable when the heads of bones were broken or capsular ligaments were torn.[24] When the fracture involved the skull, the danger posed to the brain by excessive pressure was well-recognized, and the 18th century surgeon was more than prepared to trephine at the drop of a hat.

In the event of an amputation two or more surgeon's mates would hold the patient down on the procedure table for the duration. The patient was probably conscious and capable of providing illuminating character descriptions for those doing the restraining. A leather tourniquet would be placed four fingers above the line where the offending limb was to be removed. Then with the dexterity of a master swordsman, the surgeon would whip out his amputation knife and slice through the soft tissue down to the bone of the damaged limb. Arteries spurting blood were strategically moved aside by tacking them away from the main area with crooked needles. A leather retractor was then placed on the bone and pulled back to allow the surgeon a clear field of operation. Then the surgeon would choose either his small bone saw to remove arms or a large

---

[24] The Evolution of Forward Surgery in the US Army: From the Revolutionary War. Edited by Lance P. Steahly, David W. Cannon (Sr.).

upper femur saw to remove a leg above the knee. A competent surgeon could saw through the bone in less than forty-five seconds. Speed was of the essence as arteries were buried in tissue skin flapped over and sutured. Bandages with pure white linen cloth and a wool cap were placed on the stump. The patient, who had more than likely gone into shock and had a much lower than normal temperature, was stabilized when possible. The survival rate for this procedure was a meager 35 percent.

Dr. John Jones was one of the most important Continental Army surgeons of the day and a staunchly conservative patriot who stated the obvious when he urged that surgeons acquire as much learning and training as possible. He earned his M.D. at Rheims before moving on to Paris to study under the auspices of eminent French surgeons. There were a surprising variety of surgical procedures available to 18th century surgeons such as lithotomy, (cutting out bladder stones), setting of fractures, reduction of dislocations, and amputations, which were very common.

The skill with which Dr. Jones was able to perform lithotomies when he returned from his training abroad reduced some of the trepidation that patients felt at the prospect of being the subject of any potential surgical intervention. Dr. Jones was reported to be able to perform a lithotomy in three minutes. On occasion, using a lateral perineal approach, he completed the procedure in one minute and a half. This was quite impressive but nothing really new because the ancient art of lithotomy was first noted by the Greeks (who knew a thing or two about getting rid of stones, but more about them later). The fact that some continental surgeons knew how to remove a fistula was thanks to France's King Louis XIV. On one occasion he was being a terrible pain in the derriere because of the nagging pain in his own derriere. French surgeons, sweating profusely and probably under great duress, successfully conducted surgery in 1686 to remove his majesty's royal anal fistula.[25] The excellent result of this surgical intervention inspired confidence both in the surgeons and the actual

---

[25] Progress in Proctology: Proceedings of the 3rd International Congress of Hedrologicum Conlegium. Edited by J. Hoferichter (Erlangen-Nuremberg, Germany, Springer Science & Business Media, 1968).

procedure. British surgeon William Cheselden[26] who greatly impressed his fellow practitioners with his dexterity, had performed the successful removal of a cataract. There was a lot of knowledge out there; however, the problem was general agreement regarding applicable curatives and treatments.

It was entirely possible that some of the medical officers assigned to each Continental regiment had served their apprenticeships with a qualified physician or surgeon rather than having experienced a formal education. They received abominably small remuneration for their services, and it was alleged that to supplement their low pay they often dipped into the funds provided to purchase medicine and supplies. At the start of the war, there were three thousand five hundred physicians and surgeons living in America, but only four hundred of them had actual medical degrees of any description.

In 1756, the post of Inspector of Regimental Infirmaries was established to ensure that professional standards were maintained, that money collected was properly accounted for, and that the patients received proper care. It was a move in the right direction. The Revolutionary War would highlight the necessity to have trained physicians and surgeons in their ranks. Some of them would become legends in their own right.

---

[26] The Anatomy of the Human Body. By William Cheselden.

CHAPTER THREE

The Overtures of 1812

The official end of the American Revolution on September 3, 1783, resulted in a peace treaty signed by all belligerents. After this date, plans were made to close the hospitals that had been caring for wounded Continental Army soldiers. It is generally assumed that the medical board, which was formed the previous summer, was faced with the decision whether to transfer the "invalids and debilitated men" remaining in the Army to the Invalid Corps, or completely discharge them from the Army and determine their eligibility for a pension. The remaining members of the Continental Hospital Department functioned for a while as a peacetime organization dedicated to the care of these men at West Point, Albany, and Philadelphia. By the summer of 1783, General George Washington was contemplating closing the department by the following summer. Those still remaining in Continental Army service were officially made redundant June 2, 1784. Before anyone had the temerity to ask, "What are we going to do now?" Congress decided to abandon its reliance on state militias and increase the size of the Regular Army to 10,000 men.

On March 2, 1799, it created another medical department to regulate the "Medical Establishment" of all the armed forces. Congress appointed an official physician-general responsible for all military hospitals and all medical and surgical practices or services concerning the army and navy of the United States. They also appointed an apothecary-general, a purveyor responsible for providing medical stores, and a competent number of hospital surgeons to complete the set up.

When it came to their altruistic considerations of veterans, the American Congress was way ahead of its European counterparts. In 1802, Congress established standards for the Regular Army that included invalid pensions for totally disabled officers. This payment would amount to roughly one-half of the monthly soldiers pay, and all enlisted personnel (regardless of grade) would get five dollars per month. Orphans (under age sixteen) and widows of commissioned officers who died in service as a consequence of wounds received half pay for five years. These provisions were generally extended to troops recruited to fight in the War of 1812, the Indian Wars, and the ensuing Mexican War.

In 1805, Congress recognized the fact that some disabilities might develop years after the fact and consequently provided compensation for what today we commonly refer to as "service-connected disabilities." In 1806, Congress completed the federalization of invalid pensions by assuming responsibility for all those who fought the "common enemy," also known as the British. This included "all volunteers, militia, state troops." and basically anyone who would pick up a musket and fire it in the general direction of the British.

By the beginning of the 19th century, Military medicine appeared to be in considerably better condition than it had been at any time throughout the previous millennia. Triage, trauma care, and military public health were still embryonic, but positive progress had been made. While this evolution occurred in Europe as well as in North America, a lot of knowledge was gained from the experiences of surgeons and physicians who had fought in the Napoleonic Wars.

The British may have relinquished most of their colonies in North America, but they were still allied with Native American tribes in the Northwest Territories (Illinois, Indiana, Ohio, Michigan, and Wisconsin). At a time when most places in America were named after the last Native American to leave or the first white man to arrive, several tribes populated the Northwest Territories. These included the Shawnee, Kickapoo, Sauk, Fox, and Winnebago. They formed a Native American confederacy led by Shawnee prophet Tenskwatawa and his brother Tecumseh[27] that had arisen to contest U.S. settlement in the territory. In a concerted effort to halt U.S. westward expansion the British actively supported this confederacy. They thought it wise to protect British interests in Canada by creating a Native American buffer state between U.S. territory and British Canada. This would be something akin to the country of Belgium, which was established to create a buffer state between France and the Netherlands and is often rightfully referred to as a geographic wedgie. Congress considered the mere suggestion of a buffer state objectionable, and the proposal was received like a digestive malady in a confined space. These were the main reasons that war erupted between the United States and Great Britain in 1812.

It is, however, fair to state that when Congress declared war on Great Britain on June 18, 1812, it was militarily and medically unprepared. It took a full nine months and a considerable number of meetings before Congress reestablished the posts of physician, surgeon, and apothecary general. All the departments would work together in concert. The militias were already relatively self-sufficient and provided their own surgeons while the Regular Army provided medical supplies.

The Medical Department was slow to expand, and the newly established medical districts operated autonomously. Friction between the regimental surgeons and those at the general hospitals exacerbated the problems. On the northern frontier with Canada, where much of the action occurred, disease was decimating some units, causing one commander to report that the troops were suffering badly since they had taken up positions on the border. At the time surgical intervention was kept to the minimum because of the limited knowledge of anatomy, scant knowledge

---

27 Tecumseh and the Prophet: The Shawnee Brothers Who Defied a Nation. Peter Cozzens Diversified Publishing, 15 Sep 2020.

of bacteriology, fear of infection, and lack of viable anesthetics. In the Northern Military District, twelve thousand patients were admitted to military hospitals, but only a meager seven operations were conducted, two of which were amputations.

The most enduring lesson the United States Army learned from the War of 1812 was how the Army Medical Department desperately needed to be restructured. Even though Regimental surgeons were not officially part of the department, they were required to submit monthly reports to the Physician General and Surgeon General, and starting in 1815 regimental surgeons were tasked with the training other medical candidates. It took a while, but eventually hospital hygiene and sanitation improved quite dramatically. The permanent peacetime Army Medical Department was established in 1818 under the auspices of the then-Secretary of War John C. Calhoun.

One particular surgeon the War of 1812, W. E. Horner,[28] wrote a series of articles on the surgical cases he had encountered and the conclusions he had drawn from them. He remarked that buckshot wounds could bring tears of pain to the recipient but rarely proved dangerous. Another means of suppressing levity were the capacious English musket balls that Horner believed that made amputation an absolutely necessity rather than an option, particularly when one of the "large cylindrical bones was hit." Horner was very familiar with French surgeon Dr. Dominique Jean Larrey's (1766–1842) preference for immediate amputation, and credited or blamed him with the preference Americans displayed in favor of early surgical intervention.

There were instances during the War of 1812 when the survival rate among prospective amputees whose impending amputations were temporarily postponed was higher than those whose surgery was performed soon after the wound was inflicted. The onset of hot weather greatly decreased the patient's chances for survival of a major amputation due to the increased risk of infection and mortification. Muscle tissue had a tendency to retract to an unusual degree during hot weather, and

---

[28] The Army Medical Department, 1775-1818. By Mary C. Gillett.

consequently many patients succumbed. Horner believed that if a patient did not have to be moved, the preferred option was to avoid inflicting the shock of amputation upon a man still suffering from the shock resulting from his wound. Indeed, if a limb had been ripped, wrenched, or blown off, Horner was in favor of letting nature take care of the situation. He said, "by her law if a bone protrudes beyond the limit of its covering by muscles and skin, she (nature) in a few weeks, reduces its length to the proper mark by the process of exfoliation."[29] Precisely what a wounded man writhing in agony with a limb hanging off wants to hear. "Good old mother nature will take care of it." Failing that, there was always the old favorite "divine intervention" to fall back on.

In 1812, Congress decided that militia and volunteer troops should have the same right to invalid pensions Regular Army soldiers enjoyed. Administration was, as always, long winded, and soldiers of the War of 1812 were no exception. Service pensions would be allocated years later, but this had been the case with service pensions for the majority of those who had served in the Revolutionary War. Some could say, "If it's worth having, it's worth waiting for," but this would be scant compensation for the peg leg, or those invalided in the service of their young nation.

On March 3, 1813, while the Regular. Army's general staff were reorganizing, Congress created the positions of Physician, Surgeon General, and Apothecary General, with the condition that these positions would be allocated to civilians. The main difference between the new order and the existing department established in 1799 was that this new organization only involved the army, and attributed ultimate responsibility for specific duties to President James Madison. The new regulations prohibited the conducting of private practice to all army physicians and charted the specific duties of the Physician and the Surgeon General. This reorganization entailed specific details regarding the tasks of nurses and the use of provisions and medicines purchased for the Medical Department. On June 11, 1813, the position of Physician and Surgeon General of the Medical Department was given to Revolutionary War veteran and

---

[29] The Army Medical Department, 1775-1818. By Mary C. Gillett.

notable eccentric Dr. James Tilton. He may have been a few sandwiches short of a good picnic on occasion, but he successfully organized one of the first American treaties on military medicine, and he had experience in military hospitals and expanded knowledge on the prevention and cure of diseases relating to the Army.

During that pivotal year there was military activity in both the North and the South of the United States. General Andrew Jackson successfully led his Tennessee units against the Creek Indians of the Mississippi Territory, which culminated the following year at the Battle of Horseshoe Bend. It devastated the Creek nation and their number was reduced by approximately 15 percent. Jackson was preparing to ethnically cleanse the whole area in preparation for white expansion. When the Creek nation was forced to sign "The Treaty of Fort Jackson," they had to surrender twenty-three million acres of land and solemnly promise to never again ally with the British or Spanish against the Americans. The defeat of the Creek nation was punitive and ultimately destructive.

While Jackson ethnically cleansed the Mississippi region, General William Henry Harrison, commanding the Army of the Northwest was tasked with defending the American Northwest from further British encroachments. During the first siege of Fort Meigs, Harrison noted that, "There was no place to put the wounded, they lay in trenches on rails barely sufficient to keep them up out of the water, which in many places from the bleeding of the wounded, had the appearance of puddles of blood."[30] A number of his soldiers contracted "lockjaw," a spasm of the jaw muscles, causing the mouth to remain tightly closed. It is generally regarded as a typical symptom of tetanus, one of the most feared conditions caused by the Clostridium tetani bacterium, which produces a toxin that affects the brain and nervous system, leading to stiffening of the muscles. If Clostridium tetani spores reach an open wound, the neurotoxin interferes with nerves that control muscle movement. These painful muscle spasms, usually felt in the jaw and neck could severely restrict the ability to breathe, and eventually cause death.

---

[30] Kentucky in the War of 1812. By Anderson Chenault Quisenberry (Genealogical Publishing Company).

At the second siege of Fort Meigs, Shawnee warrior and diplomat Tecumseh attempted to lure the American forces into to a pitched battle with the intention of the destroying them and forcing the garrison's surrender. He failed, causing British and Native American forces to abandon the attack. Once the siege had concluded, the survivors cleared the blockhouses of stores and transformed them into temporary hospitals, but the wounded were still lacking basic provisions. The supply and distribution channels were not really working that efficiently. The situation deteriorated to such an extent that General Harrison took the initiative to place an urgent order for medicines and stores.

While America was in the process of forming a new nation, Tecumseh was attempting to unite the Indian nations living west of the Appalachian Mountains into a confederacy that would forcibly oppose further Euro-American expansionism and restrict the ethnic cleansing of Indian lands. When the War of 1812 began, Tecumseh and many of these nations had erroneously allied themselves with Britain, a constitutional monarchy with George III, a king who became known as the "mad king who lost America." Many historians attribute his mental instability to a physical genetic blood disorder called "porphyria." Its symptoms include aches and pains, as well as blue urine as depicted in the film *The Madness of King George.*

General Harrison's operations in the summer and early fall of 1813 in the Lake Erie area culminated in October with the defeat of the British and their Native American allies over the frontier in Canada at the Battle of the Thames near present day Moraviantown, Ontario. Tecumseh met his demise at this battle, which signaled the decline of united Indian resistance against the United States of America, but there would be more battles after the British were effectively dealt with.

U.S. victory and the warrior death of Tecumseh in battle abruptly ended any hope of a Native American alliance system or confederation, and the British essentially turned tail and abandoned their Native American allies who would suffer further defeats as the United States continued its westward expansion.

Virtually unknown before the war of 1812, after his victory against the British at the Battle of New Orleans in 1814, Andrew Jackson became a national hero. The Battle of New Orleans occurred after the Treaty of Ghent[31] had been signed and sealed to end hostilities—but it hadn't been delivered. If only they would have had email. The treaty formally ended the war, but ultimately proved that very little had actually been achieved because there was no significant change in pre-war borders or boundaries. In accordance with the terms of the treaty, the British returned nearly four thousand Americans who had been classified as prisoners of war and pressed into British service. The end of hostilities ushered in the "Era of Good Feelings,"[32] during which time American-British relations improved significantly. The British completely forgot about the defeats and the Native Americans who had supported them were left to their fate.

When Andrew Jackson became president, he would personally condone ethnic cleansing and supervise further relocation of Native Americans, ultimately resulting in the destruction of tens of thousands of lives, and an entire way of life that had existed centuries before the arrival of the first white settlers was in danger of being completely eradicated.

After their defeat at the Battle of New Orleans and as British soldiers crossed the Atlantic, another campaign was underway in the lowlands of Europe. They wouldn't arrive in time but this campaign would conclude with the terrifying Battle of Waterloo, where there was an American officer present who would have also experienced the carnage at close range.

New York-born Col. Sir William Howe De Lancey was a highly respected friend of Sir Arthur Wellesley, the Duke of Wellington (aka The Iron Duke), and remained in relatively close proximity to the great man throughout the battle on the day of his greatest triumph. On the afternoon of the battle, mounted on horseback and talking to Wellington, he was knocked clean from his horse when struck in the back by a spent cannon ball. The initial impact shattered eight of De Lancey's ribs. While the battle still raged, a Lieutenant of the 1st Foot Guards witnessed the

---

31 Treaty of Ghent of 1814 with Great Britain. By Theodore Lyman.

32 The Economy of Early America: Historical Perspectives & New Directions. By Cathy D. Matson (Penn State Press).

event and ordered four soldiers to carry the wounded officer to the safety of a barn at Mont-Saint-Jean just behind the allied lines, which had been requisitioned as a temporary aid station by the British and allies.

After the battle, Wellesley erroneously announced De Lancey's death in his dispatches. When the Duke discovered his mistake, he immediately rode to Mont-Saint-Jean where De Lancey was being tended. Wellesley told De Lancey of his error, and even joked with his old friend, "Why, De Lancey! You will know what your friends said of you after you were dead," to which Sir William bravely replied, "I hope I shall."[33]

He was buried on June 28, 1815, in a cemetery in St. Josse-ten-Noode, on the south side of the Chaussée de Louvain. In 1889, by order of her majesty Queen Victoria, De Lancey's remains, and those of other officers who fell at Waterloo, were moved to a massive monument in Evere, a suburb of Brussels near the present-day headquarters of NATO.

Many historians assumed that De Lancey had died in the barn at Mont-Saint-Jean, due to its well-documented role as a British hospital during and after the battle. But doubts remained, and other details of De Lancey's last days were shrouded in mystery. In 1999, in a corner of an attic, Lady Magdalene's great, great, great grandson made a startling discovery. Inside a dust-covered trunk, he found the widowed bride's original diary, two portraits of young Magdalene, and forty hand-signed letters.

Magdalene rushed from Antwerp with exceptional haste to see her ailing husband. Accompanied by a certain Mr. Hay, she noted in her letters that she rode in a carriage through packed crowds of wounded, past fields filled with the dead from the battle that made their horses "scream at the smell of corruption." Magdalene describes her emotion as she waited to see whether her husband was still alive: "How fervently and sincerely I resolved that if I saw him alive for one hour I never would repine! I had almost lost my recollection, with the excess of anxiety and

---

[33] A Week at Waterloo In 1815: Lady de Lancey's Narrative: Being an Account of How She Nursed Her Husband, Colonel Sir William Howe de Lancey, Quartermaster-General of the Army, Mortally Wounded in the Great Battle. By Lady Magdalene De Lancey (Creative Media Partners, LLC, 2018).

suspense, when Mr. Hay called out, 'All's well; I have seen him. He expects you.'"[34]

She nursed Sir William for six days, until he "gave a little gulp" and shed his mortal coil. Magdalene visited her husband's grave near Brussels on July 4, 1815. "That day, three months before, I was married." Later that year, the widowed Lady Magdalene recorded her reminiscences in a journal, which was originally intended for the eyes of her close friends and family. She may have felt the need to protect her reputation as a devoted and grieving wife, but malicious rumors circulated that she had been insufficiently remorseful after Waterloo. She may have just been stoic, but after only being married to the man for three months, its equally possible that she didn't think her husband's passing merited the full-blown mourning routine.

Physicians and surgeons of the day owed a lot of their accumulated knowledge to the trials and errors of their predecessors, but if they had been able to look back a few thousand years, rather than a few hundred, they would have known even more. Ancient Egyptians, Greeks, and Romans had established some basic premises regarding the care of wounded soldiers and some of their potions actually worked, but precisely why they worked would remain a mystery in some cases until the present day.

---

[34] A Week at Waterloo In 1815. By Lady Magdalene De Lancey (Creative Media Partners, LLC, 2018).

CHAPTER FOUR

Egyptians, Greeks, and Romans

Physicians and surgeons that operated during the American Revolutionary War based most of their accumulated knowledge on what had been established throughout the previous centuries. It would, however, have served them well to look considerably further back at antiquity because a few thousand years before the declaration of independence, the Egyptians firmly believed that the application of successful wound treatments demanded prescribing both observable and supernatural elements. For this purpose, they would inevitably respect practical physical remedies, but be prepared to throw in the odd magic spell or spontaneous formation dance routine for added efficacy. Their medicine also relied on the combined power of incantations along with herbal concoctions to hopefully achieve a desired result. The right words could invalidate or deflect malicious forces, and the use of amulets or materials that had been in contact with powerful talismans were also expected to render a salutary effect. This was often to the detriment of the afflicted soldier whose primary consideration rarely exceeded, "Do something quick, this stings, you know?"

As punishing Middle Eastern temperatures baked the bodies of wounded, thirsty men lying prone on the field of battle, their first requirement would of course be water. One Egyptian text acknowledged that H2O served both a cosmetic and a medicinal purpose. The cosmetic application explains why both Egyptian men and women are depicted on hieroglyphics wearing what appears to be heavy eyeliner. It was actually a dark water-based substance applied around the eyes to reduce the glare of the Egyptian sun and repel flies. This ultimately implies that even when wounded soldiers were suffering badly, their eyes would still have resembled those of overtly camp female impersonators.

Whether the bullet, musket ball, arrow, or spearhead had one's name on it, it was pure chance, but being at the mercy of surgeons with dubious qualifications made soldiers a deeply superstitious lot. Lucky charms have been around as long as civilization, and Egyptian soldiers were no exception. As their troops ventured forth into battle, they often wore an amulet for protection that depicted the gruesome image of the Egyptian god Bes. This was thought to deter malevolent gods or hostile spirits of the deceased from interfering in the proceedings. In the event of Bes being preoccupied with other matters the image was augmented with a massive shield and a pair of sturdy legs that could switch direction at any given moment as the situation evolved. Ancient Egyptians didn't rely entirely on supernatural remedies when coping with physical traumas. One papyrus written during a period of internecine struggle and warfare refers to a physician actively treating battle casualties.

It describes in detail the types of weapon that would have inflicted the wounds that were used by both Egyptian soldiers and their enemies in combat. The physical treatments and prescriptions involved a compendium of substances compiled over the course of millennia. Surgery was exceedingly rare, and dissection was definitely not considered a feasible option. Physicians of the day employed a vast pharmacopoeia of natural substances such as honey and the juice of pomegranates, which served as a powerful astringent. The water lily plant that was applied to wounds and abrasions has been proven to contain analgesic properties and may also have been ingested on occasion for that purpose. Residues discovered in distinctive tall-necked vessels that may have been imported from Asia Minor suggest that there is every possibility that Egyptian physicians were acquainted with the anesthetic properties of opium. All physicians were meticulously trained and required to become skilled practitioners of physical and supernatural medicine. Some centuries later the Greeks would invoke their gods for numerous purposes, but chose to rely on more practical solutions when treating the wounded.

One passage from Homer's *Iliad* states, "A physician is worth more than several other men put together, for he can cut out arrows and spread healing herbs."[35] Bearing in mind of course, that most wounds would have resulted from the implementation of hacking, stabbing, or slashing practices employed by the incumbent ancient armies. Although their anesthetic value may have been questionable some of the "healing herbs" applied to the afflicted areas could indeed be quite efficacious.

The Ancient Greek term for the person who cared for the wounded was *iatros*, which is apparently derived from an old Ionian word meaning "extractor of arrows." The Greeks effectively cleansed wounds with a concoction assembled from wine and vinegar. Greek wine contained polyphones, which are known to be a thirty-three times more powerful bactericide than the phenols Joseph Lister used in 1865.

It's generally known that Alexander the Great's army used tourniquets made of brass and leather to staunch wounds; however they didn't have the knowledge to permanently arrest the bleeding once a tourniquet was removed. Alexander openly acknowledged the benefits of having trained physicians to accompany his powerful armies, and they operated in situations not completely alien to contemporary medical staff. He only had seven overworked physicians to tend an army of around forty thousand. His experience would inspire the Roman army to incorporate a highly organized and efficient military medical service as a standard addition to all its conquering legions.

---

[35] Neil Osterweil, "What We Can Learn From Ancient Greek Medicine," WebMD (WebMD, August 2, 2004), https://www.webmd.com/women/features/what-we-can-learn-from-ancient-greek-medicine#1.

When the Roman armies began expanding to support the imperial ambitions of their emperor, the military began to develop something that employed the protocols, which resembled a distinct system of military medicine. Once the Roman Army had defeated the Greeks and forced them to renounce independence by incorporating their territories into their empire, the Roman medical service improved on the Greek version by incorporating trained physicians and establishing field hospitals to tend their wounded. As Plato's magnanimous phrase correctly observed, "all the good things of the conquered pass into the hands of the conquerors."

A Roman medical officer was known as the *Medicus*. This trained doctor was usually in charge of Greek or Greek-trained medical personnel known as the *Medici*. The exact rank and hierarchic position of the Medici within the army has never been conclusively ascertained. They were usually in the service of Rome after being captured as prisoners of war. Many Greek doctors would later be assuaged by fiscal considerations and even rehouse to Rome. This proves conclusively that even back then there were certain individuals in the medical profession who were easily persuaded to abandon home and hearth at the right price.

Wounded Roman soldiers would receive initial treatment by medics called *Capasarii*, who carried boxes of bandages. Later Roman army surgeons were usually given the rank of magister or "master." Records show that medical supplies and carriages for bearing the wounded were strategically placed in the middle of marching columns.

In the seventh book of Pliny's Natural History, published in 77 A.D., the author refers to Marcus Silus Ferrous Sergius,[36] Roman general and politician who lived from 218 to 201 B.C. and fought during the Punic and Epirote Wars. According to Pliny, this Roman general was one of the first soldiers to wear a prosthetic limb. The original right hand was sliced clean off in a sword fight during his second year of military service. Not only did the general live to tell the tale, undaunted, he

---

[36] The framework of an imperial legion: the fifth annual Caerleon lecture in honorem Aquilae Legionis II Augustae. By Michael Speide.

actively participated in many ensuing battles, whereupon he sustained twenty-three separate injuries to his extremities.

He managed to maintain his prowess in battle by fashioning a prosthetic iron hand capable of holding a shield and splitting enemy skulls with remarkable dexterity. His enemies were frequently reduced to awestruck silence as he stabbed, gouged, and slashed away to great effect. Twice taken prisoner by Hannibal's Carthaginians, despite being restrained in chains and shackles for months on end, he managed to escape on both occasions. Precisely how he escaped isn't documented, but it's safe to speculate that the iron hand could have had something to do with it. After he finished his military service, he ventured into the equally precarious area of public politics where he served as a Roman *Praetor*. A number of his erstwhile colleagues attempted to prevent the former general from participating in public ceremonies because of his perceived "deformity." Nevertheless, Sergius skillfully allayed his detractors, which to some extent made him the world's first advocate for the rights of veteran amputees.

In the Roman army the person who would have initially tended the general would have been the appointed Medicus, who would have had various instruments at their disposal for the treatment of wounds. The prime purpose for these instruments appears to have been the for the purpose of extraction of arrowheads and small stones fired by slings, but there were various other instruments that were remarkably similar to those employed by surgeons of the 19th and early 20th centuries. Roman surgeons used forceps, scalpels, tourniquets, ear scoops, catheters, and even arterial clamps. They wouldn't have had any real knowledge of bacterial infections, but they must have had some concept of hygiene because they usually took the precaution of boiling instruments before and after every procedure.

The Medicus had various familiar sedatives and painkillers at their disposal to enhance their bedside manner, such as opium and henbane seeds that contained scopolamine (also known as hyoscine), which is used to treat motion sickness and postoperative nausea and vomiting.

Wounded Roman soldiers were often treated with acetum, a concoction made from vinegar. It proved to be a feasible antiseptic, but by all accounts was excruciatingly painful when applied. It would take four or five Capasarii to restrain the writhing patient while the antiseptic was being liberally smeared into the wound. The recipient of their attention rarely thanked them during the procedure. The antiseptic had the capacity to prevent some infections and was even known to prevent superficial wounds from becoming fatal. Sadly, the lessons of the past were not carried on to the middle ages because most Greek and Roman information was lost to successive dynasties.

Many historians unanimously agree that the quality and effectiveness of Roman military medicine was not surpassed until at least the 17th and 18th centuries. The care given to a roman soldier was in fact almost equivalent to the care a soldier received during World War I. This has been borne out in Roman medical guides dating as far back as the 1st century A.D. Those Romans knew their stuff.

CHAPTER FIVE

I Bet That Hurts

Some of the practices indulged by those early American physicians and surgeons could even be traced back to medieval times when treatment of wounded soldiers on and off the battlefield often fell to the clergy. The imposition of stringent religious doctrine frequently impeded the quality of care received. This remained the case for many decades in the New World.

The sharp division of the medical profession into the domains of physicians and surgeons can be traced as far back as the 12th century, when the fun-loving Catholic Church officially forbade the clergy to shed blood under any circumstance. This would ultimately prove problematic after the extraction of arrowheads or crossbow bolts. Despite the restrictions priests and monks continued, often surreptitiously, to practice medicine, but actual surgery was allocated to the dubious talents of their former lay assistants, whose primary duty was shaving the monks' heads with sharp blades, and deviations on the theme. This development hailed the advent of the lower status profession of the "barber surgeon," but more about that later.

The words hospital, hospice, hospitable, etc. are derived from the Latin word *hospitale*, which was transposed to Hospitaller by the knights and their auxiliaries who adopted this suffix. The organization still exists in name to this day.

There aren't many historical references to battlefield nurses before the 18th century, but in medieval times (as in the Revolutionary War) when men took up arms, they often took their families along with them for convenience. It is, however, well documented that the women would have assumed the roles of erstwhile nurses for the wounded and dying during various historic campaigns throughout this turbulent period in history, but they would not have been afforded the title. Removing casualties from the battlefield at the time was another matter entirely. The first reference to any kind of litter used for this purpose occurs in a manuscript written around 1380.

In the late Middle Ages physicians became widely regarded as ostensibly skilled people, even if their work was based on glaringly inadequate knowledge of the human anatomy. Thanks to rigorous adherence to religious doctrine, medical experiments on dead bodies was strictly forbidden in Medieval England. Physicians charged extortionately for their services, hence only the rich could afford to pay for them. not that much has changed from then. The cures they applied could be quite bizarre, although it's fair to say that some cures, including bleeding and the use of herbs, had some logic to them even if it was very much a kind of "I bet that hurts" ersatz science. Nevertheless, it has since transpired that some of these reputedly dubious cures actually had intrinsic medicinal value.

One particular remedy allegedly invented by Saint Paul (the saint who initially harbored a seething grudge against Christians) was a potion to treat epilepsy, catalepsy, and stomach problems. The extensive list of ingredients included licorice, sage, willow, roses, fennel, cinnamon, ginger, cloves, cormorant blood, mandrake, dragon's blood, and three kinds of pepper. Although this recipe sounds more like something that would have been assembled in a witch's cauldron, precisely how reliable is the testimony of someone who claims to have procured dragons blood? Despite this some of the ingredients really do have proven medicinal value. For instance, licorice is still used to treat coughs and bronchitis. Sage is thought to improve blood flow to the brain, and willow contains salicylic acid, a component of modern-day aspirin.[37] Even though thunderous, repetitious farting was regarded more as a means of entertainment rather than a passport to social exclusion, fennel, cinnamon, and ginger are all acknowledged carminatives, treatments for relieving gas in the intestines, and colic. It is, however, doubtful that the potion would have been of any use in the treatment of epilepsy and catalepsy.

Another cure was actually known as "dragon's blood." Although dragons are frequently referred to as real beasts in several medieval texts, this product didn't pretend to be blood extracted from an actual dragon, but the bright red resin of the tree *Dracaena draco*, a species native to Morocco, Cape Verde, and the Canary Islands. Modern research has since been shown to contain significant antiseptic, antibiotic, anti-viral, and wound healing properties, and it is still used today in some parts of the world to treat dysentery.

Rubbing the slime of a snail on the affected area would be the medieval remedy for burns and scalds. Sounds like pure quackery until one discovers that it really did help to reduce blistering and ease the pain! It's been scientifically proven in recent times that snail slime contains antioxidants, antiseptic, and anesthetic along with anti-irritant, anti-inflammatory, antibiotic, and antiviral properties, as well as collagen and elastin, vital for skin repair. Combining barley with one handful of betony (grassland herb) and another handful of vervain (another herb) was a treatment for medieval headaches. Once boiled up they were wrapped in a cloth and made into a poultice that would be firmly placed on the head of the sufferer to relieve the symptoms, which it inevitably did, but it also restricted certain widely-practiced procreative activities. At least the wearer of the said poultice wouldn't be reduced to making the age-old excuse, "not tonight darling, I have a headache." Betony was used by the medieval and Tudor apothecary as an ingredient in remedies

---

[37] Medieval Herbal Remedies: The Old English Herbarium and Anglo-Saxon Medicine. By Anne Van Arsdall.

to be taken internally for all kinds of ailments, as well as in poultices for external use, as in this case.

Modern medicine still makes use of the alkaloid drugs found in betony for treating severe headaches and migraine and "Vervain's glycoside" (a class of molecules in which a sugar molecule is bonded to a "non-sugar" molecule) derivatives too are used in modern treatments for migraine, depression, and anxiety. It was alleged that vervain was used to stem the flow of blood from Christ's wounds during his crucifixion. It might have proved more useful when the crown of thorns was placed on the poor man's head, but that's the beauty of hindsight. So even though the physicians were referred to as "quacks," it has transpired that medieval medicine wasn't all blatant quackery.

Notable surgeons John Bradmore and Thomas Morstede were both dedicated surgeons employed during the Wars of the Roses by the Lancastrian Kings Henry IV and Henry V, respectively. Bradmore put his own life on the line when he played an integral and memorable part in saving the life of the man who would eventually become Henry V. The same one celebrated and famed by Shakespeare for his victory against the French at Agincourt. Prince Henry was only sixteen years old at the time of the battle.

Once upon a time during the Wars of the Roses at the Battle of Shrewsbury, the then-young Prince Henry, Prince of Wales, was hit square in the face by an arrow. Precisely which weapon was used to launch the offending projectile isn't known, but although Bradmore consistently refers to it as an arrow, the depth of penetration achieved by this particular projectile suggests that it was probably fired from a crossbow. Crossbow bolts are relatively short. The main differences between an arrow and a bolt are its flight characteristics. While a longbow arrow's parabolic arc of fall depends on the lift gained in flight, bolts fall at the same rate, and can be fired directly at an intended target. Moreover, the circumference of a crossbow bolt shaft is marginally wider than that of an arrow. The four-sided bolt head could penetrate armor with relative ease.

It was during a troubled and turbulent time in "Merry Olde England" at the Battle of Shrewsbury during the Wars of the Roses when Lancastrian King Henry IV's ferocious army squared off against a rebel alliance led by Sir Henry "Hostpur" Percy, the Earl of Worcester, and the Earl of Douglas. Eyewitness accounts claim that archers fired so vigorously that the sky turned black and the missiles cut down the royal vanguard "like apples fallen in the autumn." What transpired was one of the most remarkable cases of battlefield surgery that occurred in the Middle Ages.

Appointed head surgeon John Bradmore was a man working under increasingly insurmountable duress. The primary reason for his consternation was because he possessed little more than a basic rudimentary knowledge of cranial anatomy. Bradmore had examined a few severed heads, which were relatively easy to procure at the time for obvious reasons, but the future King's head was another matter entirely.

As Bradmore carefully, extremely carefully examined the prince he noticed that the bolt head had penetrated to a depth of six inches and was firmly lodged in the rear of the prince's skull like the sword in the stone. This was one occasion when the Hippocrates "humors" were of no value. A narrow eight-inch pole lodged in one's face was not conducive to the prince's humor.

The wound would have bled profusely for a start. That well-known English reserve was prodigiously abandoned as frantic attempts were made to remedy the situation. Unfortunately, all the attempts did was subject his stricken majesty to further agonizing pain and induce him to vociferously accuse Bradmore of being of uncertain parentage, or something to that effect.

But necessity is indeed the mother of invention and the prince's protestations induced the understandably worried surgeon, who was under extreme duress, to devise an ingenious extraction plan to remove the arrowhead. According to one version of the events, Bradmore cleverly improvised a pair of hollow tongs that were the width of an arrowhead with a screw-like thread at the end of each arm and a separate screw mechanism running through the center. Much to the chagrin of the prince, who was at this stage somewhat lost for intelligible words, the wound had to be enlarged and deepened before the tongs could be effectively inserted.

This was eventually achieved by means of large and long probes made from "pith of old elder stitched with purified linen cloth infused with rose honey." The arrow entered at an angle (ex traverso), and after the arrow shaft was extracted, the arrowhead remained in the furthermost part of the bone of the skull for the depth of six inches.[38]

When Bradmore determined that he had reached the bottom of the wound, he cautiously inserted the ad hoc tongs at the same angle as the arrow had entered. The screw finally latched onto the arrowhead and, he wrote, "by moving it to and fro, little by little (with the help of God) I extracted the arrowhead."

He maneuvered the instrument into the socket of the arrowhead. Bradmore even had the acumen to attempt to prevent infection by treating the wounds with white wine. The alcohol would have inadvertently served as a kind of disinfectant. After the wound was cleansed, he packed it with wads of flax (linen) soaked in cleansing ointment, infused with an unlikely combination of bread, sops, barley, honey, and turpentine oil. As the wound healed, he reduced the amount of packing every two days until twenty days after the battle he able to confidently report that "the wound was perfectly well cleansed." This was remarkably fortuitous for Bradmore, who had saved the prince and himself from a fate worse than death.

Prince Henry, Prince of Wales, recovered completely and when he became Henry V, he went on to conduct the famed "Agincourt Campaign." Bradmore died in 1412 and was replaced by Thomas Morstede. At this juncture in history the pace quickens a little, and Morstede is allowed, nay positively encouraged in fact, to assemble an entourage of surgeons, apprentices, and medical men. Certain individuals regard this collective as being one of the first professional medical corps to accompany an English fighting force. The quasi surgical intervention performed by John Bradmore might explain why contemporary portraits of the King always show him in profile from the left side, never revealing what is on

---

[38] https://wilson.fas.harvard.edu/stigma-in-shakespeare/henry-v%E2%80%99s-face-in-early-english-literature.

the right side of his face, which may have been somewhat disfigured by scars from the wound.

The church was unquestioningly all-powerful and constantly reminded medieval peasants that all illness was a punishment from God for sinful behavior. So apart from the odd happy heathen, the milling throngs zealously believed this. Therefore, any illness was self-imposed, and a direct result of the individual's sinful ways. It's entirely possible that Morstede or Bradmore, or both of these surgeons, possessed the forbidden knowledge vehemently restricted by the religious hierarchy, but in line with the assertions of Hippocrates, war and conflict remained the archetypal learning ground for many medical innovations. Some of these discoveries have had a significant impact on our understanding of the body and the devastating impact of the battlefield trauma on both mind and body. The paradox was that while medical staff devised and initiated new methods of treatment, the combatants developed deadly new ways to maim and murder, which in turn presented new challenges to the medical community.

Gunpowder, which was widely available during the French and Indian War and the American Revolutionary War, had been employed for various purposes for a few centuries in the Far East before it reached the European mainland. Its invention was reputedly established around 850 A.D. as the result of Chinese alchemists attempting to find a potion that perpetuated longevity. Maybe these alchemists were doing precisely that when the COVID-19 virus escaped, if indeed it was manufactured. If you pay attention to people with too much power and horrendously bad hairstyles, then it was a foregone conclusion.

The alchemists soon discovered that gunpowder was an extremely volatile substance, and regarding the prolongation of longevity, its ad hoc discovery probably had the reverse effect, but this has never been officially ascertained. There's every possibility that it could have been used experimentally before this time, but it doesn't appear to have had any significant presence in European armies and battles until the 15th century.

Numerous armies had already used incendiary materials to deter potential assailants for hundreds of years. The most notorious concoction was known as "Greek Fire" and many writers of antiquity refer to flaming arrows, fire pots, and the use of such substances as pitch, naphtha, sulfur, and charcoal. The substance could be thrown in pots or discharged mortar-like from tubes whereupon it apparently caught fire spontaneously and could not be extinguished with water.

Consequently, various treatments for serious burns were also available. Hippocrates had recommended the use of bulky dressings impregnated with rendered pig fat and resin with alternated warm vinegar soaks, augmented with tanning solutions made from oak bark. In the 1st century AD Celsus, a Greek philosopher and ardent opponent of early Christianity prescribed a burn lotion, which had bacteriostatic properties and consisted of wine and myrrh. One of the simplest and still used methods of treating burns was recommended around 900, by Rhases (Muhammad ibn Zakariya al-Razi) an Arabian physician of some distinction, who sagely suggested dousing the afflicted part or parts in cold water. The simple ideas were often the best ones.

By the 16th century A.D., battlefield surgeons such as previously mentioned André Paré began to make their appearance in French armies. As the feudal system dissipated in Europe and nations began to take shape, Europeans subsequently formed armies to defend themselves, and on occasion conquer new territory. With the new nations also came a rebirth (renaissance) of learning. In contrast to their western counterparts (the Arab and Byzantine cultures that retained many ancient Greek and Roman texts), European medicine was slow to pick up on this until the texts were translated and reintroduced into medical practice. Unfortunately, some of the medical texts were lost in translation, which resulted in improper treatment of certain injuries. For example, infection was often introduced into wounds in the belief that infection assisted in healing despite Greek and Roman physicians understanding that this was a wholly erroneous concept.

The introduction of gunpowder to the battlefield in the late middle ages meant that surgeons had to adapt their techniques accordingly. They discovered that lead balls fired from smoothbore muskets had the potential to inflict horrific wounds, particularly when they passed through arms and legs. Compound fractures, which were rare in ancient times, became commonplace due to the force of the bullet or projectile hitting a bone. Although most combatants would survive the initial injuries sustained by gunfire, there were inevitably other complications that would develop and prove ultimately fatal.

During the Seven Years' War and the Revolutionary War, among other muskets available at the time the British military employed their own Brown Bess musket, which had been introduced in 1722 and remained standard issue until sometime around 1838. In the hands of a trained infantryman, it was capable of firing approximately three rounds per minute. The Brown Bess Musket was a flintlock musket, it would use flint in order to spark the gunpowder loaded into the gun to cause the gun to fire. It took precisely twenty actions to load and reload the musket, so three shots a minute was no mean feat.

The primary problem for many injuries inflicted by musket balls was that of infection. Nearly all gunshot wounds became infected either due to the nature of the injury itself or due to filthy clothing, dirt, and other contaminated material being forced into the wound when the body was impacted by the musket ball or piece of shrapnel. The situation would be further exacerbated by the dubious personal hygiene of the wounded and the unsanitary conditions they would have to endure following injury. It didn't help that the surgeon probing for the musket ball or shrapnel had unwashed, detritus ridden fingers and hands. In an effort to promote healing, there was often a high risk of death from infection rather than from the injury itself.

Personal hygiene was indeed a serious problem, and the standards of hygiene the Pilgrims brought with them from the Old World was severely lacking. They didn't regard washing as the main ingredient for cleanliness, early Americans focused their sanitary regimens around linen, of all things, but there is sufficient evidence to suggest that most people washed at least one a week whether they needed it or not. Despite the strict religious doctrines, the Pilgrims didn't regard cleanliness as being next to Godliness. While the poor would bathe innocuously in streams, rivers, and lakes, the more affluent members of society would congregate in notorious bathhouses. Back in the Old World the Catholic Church vehemently disapproved of bathhouses, and surprisingly enough, their vociferous objections were not entirely groundless. Many of these places were surreptitiously, and in some cases openly, used as brothels.

As the centuries passed, personal hygiene considerations actually deteriorated to such an extent that by the 17th century bathing was positively frowned upon. Consequently, people stank to the high heavens, and this would remain the case until advent of the Industrial Revolution in the mid–18th century and the discovery of the germ theory of disease in the second half of the 19th century. Until that time hygiene and sanitation were not universally accepted as the reasons behind some illnesses and diseases such as cholera and typhoid.

From the late middle ages and for many ensuing centuries, the only ubiquitously acknowledged way of dealing with an afflicted limb was immediate amputation. The problem was that the surgeon's skill and dexterity wouldn't necessarily be assessed on his knowledge of medicine but on precisely how fast they could remove the offending limb. It's almost comforting to acknowledge that although the name had an entirely different connotation, "despicable hackers" were around even then. Despite the advent of gunpowder and shot, the ingenuity and amazing capacity of ad hoc medical staff to adapt techniques and improvise while under fire saved countless lives in often horrific circumstances. The techniques developed in combat by surgeons such as Morstede, Bradmore, and Paré would resound and disseminate throughout the world of medicine and remain with us right up to the present day.

Ambroise Paré[39] was one of the primary innovators of what we have come to regard as "battlefield medicine." He served as royally appointed military surgeon for a number of French Kings. He began his career, not surprisingly, as an apprentice barber before joining the army in 1536, where he was gainfully employed for the ensuing thirty years. These barber-surgeons were (on occasion) skilled workers who apart from being

---

[39] Ten Books of Surgery with the Magazine of the Instruments Necessary for it. By Ambroise Pare (Author), Robert White Linker (Translator), Nathan Womack (Translator) (2010).

able to provide a suitable trim and a shave were trained by apprenticeship to perform basic surgical and other medical procedures. Young apprentices often trained under skilled barber-surgeons in the army and many remained with the army even after mastering the trade. Paré is widely acknowledged as someone who pioneered modern battlefield wound treatment and radically improved on existing techniques designed for the treatment of war wounds.

Movies depicting the treatment of battlefield wounds in centuries past often depict a white-hot sword or dagger being skillfully applied to cauterize and seal the affected area. The viewer is usually treated to the cringe worthy sound of searing flesh and agonized howls of derision from the reluctant patient. For centuries, tissue exposed following an amputation would indeed be cauterized this way. Searing the open wound often did little to stop the bleeding and the procedure itself was so terribly painful that many patients expired on the table from shock. Paré tried using ligatures to staunch post-operative bleeding. Using this technique, open arteries would be tied off using thread. The ensuing infection caused by these ligatures also had the potential to cause death, but his pioneering work has been widely acknowledged as a veritable milestone in medicine.

Another common, but equally painful method of treating open wounds was the practice of pouring boiling oil onto the afflicted area. On one occasion Paré had exhausted his personal supply, so he combined a tincture made from egg yolk, turpentine, and oil of roses. The following morning, he was astounded to see that all the soldiers who had been treated with his tincture were in a considerably better condition than those who had been subjected to the excruciating boiling oil treatment. According to witnesses the latter had a tendency to smell like something that resembled a pan full of cooked bacon but didn't excite the gastric juices or promise a cure for a powerful hangover.

Paré remained receptive to new ideas, such as those proposed by Flemish-born anatomist Andreas Vesalius, the man who in 1543 published his book *De Humani Corporis Fabrica*.[40] The book's contents were

---

40   De Humani Corporis Fabrica. By Andreas Vesalius (Norman Publishing).

unprecedented and based largely on the results of his personal observations of human dissection. It transformed anatomy into a subject that relied on annotations taken directly from these dissections as opposed to the perpetual guessing game employed by many barber surgeons of the day.

Paré was a pioneering exponent of anatomy-based treatments that introduced the implantation of teeth, artificial limbs, and artificial eyes made of gold and silver, among other things. He invented many scientific instruments, popularized the use of the truss for hernia, and was the first to suggest syphilis as a cause of aneurysm (swelling of blood vessels), along with introducing revolutionary new ideas in obstetrics. He also reintroduced the ligature of arteries instead of cauterization and designed an early version of a modern hemostat, which rendered the amputation of larger limbs and made it a more acceptable procedure. By 1545, Paré had collected enough knowledge on the subject of battlefield medicine to publish a book titled *The Method of Curing Wounds Caused by Arquebus and Firearms.* He was a true innovator who expertly engendered the methods of care of battlefield trauma wounds.

His famed work as a war surgeon, and afterward as a surgeon in Paris, together with the publication of his book Les Oeuvres in 1575, ensured that Ambroise Paré's techniques and ideas were disseminated across the whole of Europe. His success was also influential in initiating the rise in status of the previously feared barber surgeons.

During the French and Indian War and the Revolutionary War a battle wound would qualify the injured for bullet extractors, bone saws, and even skull elevators. Anesthetics still hadn't been developed, and some of the cures such as repetitive bleeding actually worsened the predicament of the sufferers. Bloodletting or phlebotomy, usually performed with the assistance of leeches, was based on an ancient system of medicine in which blood and other bodily fluids were regarded as "humors" that had to remain in proper balance to maintain health. In either war, there was no shortage of wounded personnel to practice on. Musket balls, cannons, typhus, and dysentery took their toll, but it's surprising how many survived frequently horrific injuries.

Medical innovations were increasing, and although there was still a long way to go before the advent of bactericides, at least efforts were being undertaken to recognize and deal with the physical maladies that beset soldiers in combat.

By 1718, French surgeon Jean Louis Petit[41] had invented a screw tourniquet to control bleeding. The screw tourniquet made thigh amputations possible and reduced the risks associated with amputations below the knee. The screw tourniquet was still widely in use during the American Civil War. As amputations became safer, military surgeons gave greater emphasis to preparing limbs for prosthesis. Flap and lateral incision amputations became common procedures. Despite this, the death rate from amputation remained high for the duration until methods were developed in the 19th century to control infection and shock.

---

[41] L'art de guerier les maladies des os etc. By Jean Louis Petit.

CHAPTER SIX

Are We There Yet?

The word "nurse" is derived from the Latin word *nutrire*, meaning to suckle, and in that case probably referred to a maternity nurse. This was probably because women were regarded as such lowly creatures in the misogynistic middle ages that they weren't really regarded as being fit for many purposes, apart from child bearing and providing for men both horizontally and vertically. It wasn't until the late 16th century that the word "nurse" obtained it's contemporary meaning as someone who provides care and comfort for the infirm. Nevertheless, the earliest references to nurses are strictly in the male domain, and they occur long before male nurses became the norm. The word alone is a noun and a verb and unless a gender prefix is used, the noun remains an androgynous reference. Nursing became much more popularized in Europe during the Middle Ages, due primarily to its spread by the all-powerful Catholic Church.

After a lot of the hospital establishments fell into disrepair, Emperor Charlemagne decided to restore and equip them with all of the latest medical equipment of that time. The Emperor also demanded that hospitals should be attached to every cathedral and monastery within Europe, which helped to stimulate a popular demand for even more nurses.

Monasteries began situating hospitals within their premises, as well as building separate infirmaries, with the stipulation that these services were only available to the genuinely pious. Heathens and those of other religions were not welcome.

Before female nurses were recognized as the caring individuals we know today, their contributions were restricted by harsh conventionally stereotyped categories. They were expected to be loving wives whose deep attachments to their sick or wounded husbands helped them to transcend the religiously-motivated natural revulsion to their gender. Or they were asexual nuns, serving God as well as soldiers. They may have even been the ill reputed and maligned "camp followers," women whose willingness to nurse for pay often transposed them into disreputable objects of derision. Either way, women nurses were not referred to with any recognizable contemporary reverence until the mid–18th century.

As previously mentioned, many soldiers still took their women and children to war with them, which meant that a substantial part of an army's baggage train was simply an accumulation of itinerant households. The women in the train were subject to military justice, and they were required to help fortify camps. Soldiers and officers who attempted to exempt their female dependents from this type of work caused great consternation among their fellow officers and troops. As a rule, the women and the whole train of non-combatants were under the surveillance of an officer who was disparagingly referred to as the *Hurenwaibel* (overseer of whores).

It was thanks to such derogatory references and a wide variety of other reasons that during the late 17th century, nursing as a reputable métier dissipated. In the United Kingdom during the Protestant reformation most monasteries were shut down along with the hospitals they housed. The nuns that had been working as nurses were forced to leave the profession and stay at home. This caused a general stagnation in the profession between the 17th and 18th centuries in Europe, except in areas where the Catholic religion held sway, but even there the role of nurses decreased quite dramatically along with their numbers.

This inspired the ones who wished to remain practicing to diversify and develop new services such as offering care as erstwhile community nurses to those within the estate of their patrons. While these nurses resided at the estate, they would be required to perform a myriad of tasks typically undertaken by apothecaries, physicians, and surgeons. While nursing faced more tumultuous times during the years to come, the demand for nurses actually increased along with the almost reverential preference by the public to be treated by a caring nurse as opposed to a dangerous doctor. Medical care in the 18th and early 19th centuries was still embryonic, but there were some doctors and surgeons who were making others in their profession sit up and take notice. One such doctor was Dominique Jean Larrey.

CHAPTER SEVEN

Napoleon's Hero

After the cataclysmic Battle of Borodino on September 7, 1812, Dr. Dominique Jean Larrey performed over two hundred amputations, each one conducted with consummate skill and speed, which procured effusive praise from his boss Napoleon Bonaparte, Emperor of France. It's safe to say that Larrey was one of the true pioneers of battlefield surgery and a primary exponent of the hitherto neglected "humanitarian" approach. Some notables have described Larrey as the true father of modern military surgery, and even by today's standards he is considered as the model military surgeon. The "Triage" system[42] originally introduced by Larrey has saved thousands of lives, from the American Civil War to the Iraq and Afghanistan wars.

Larrey accompanied Napoleon Bonaparte throughout almost eighteen years that incorporated twenty-five campaigns, sixty battles, and more than four hundred military engagements. Doctors such as Dominique Jean Larrey[43] played an integral part in recognizing and en-

---

[42] Emergency Care. By Susan H. Gray (Cherry Lake).
[43] Relation Historique Et Chirurgicale de l'Expédition de l'Armée d'Orient, En Egypte Et En Syrie. By Dominique Jean Larrey (Creative Media Partners, LLC).

dorsing the value of well-trained nurses on the battlefield. Larrey became Napoleon's personal favorite.

In 1787 he was appointed surgeon to the French royal navy and participated in a cruise to the North American waters, visiting Newfoundland as a surgeon on the frigate Vigilante; however, he soon had to resign because of chronic seasickness and returned to Paris where he worked as aide chirurgien L'Hôtel-Dieu and as field surgeon at Les Invalides. By 1790, he had established himself as assistant Senior Surgeon at Les Invalides.

Admired by his American contemporaries, he has been described by many notables as the true father of modern military surgery. The number of procedures and body parts that have been named after the great man validates the significance of Larrey's work. He was responsible for among other things the amputation at the shoulder joint known as "Larrey's amputation,". He also performed the first successful pericardiocentesis (also called pericardial tap), a medical procedure whereupon fluid is aspirated from the pericardium. Larrey also recognized the importance of ligation of the femoral artery to prevent excessive blood loss.

He was a humanitarian who urged doctors to treat the soldiers of enemy armies with dignity and compassion, and he also introduced the use of mobile medical units, which he named ambulances *volantes* ("flying ambulances") that were inspired by the Napoleonic two-wheeled gun carriages. He developed and applied the method of speedy evacuation of wounded soldiers from the battlefield during combat. Larrey spent almost eighteen years with Napoleon, accompanying him in twenty-five campaigns, sixty battles, and more than four hundred engagements.

Larrey was born on July 8, 1766, (during the reign of Louis XV) in the picturesque Campan valley of Beaudéan on the edge de l'Adour near Bagnères de Bigorre. When his father, the village cobbler, died in 1770 at the tender age of fourteen, Larrey decided not to dedicate himself to the family business. Instead, he opted for a career in medicine. His uncle Alexis Larrey who was the Chief Surgeon of the Grave Hospital at Toulouse probably inspired this decision. Uncle Alex welcomed the lad with open arms and promptly enrolled him at Esquille College that was run by a religious order known as the Brothers of the Christian Doctrine. At the end of 1787, Larrey applied and secured a position as a surgeon in the French Royal Navy. It's curious to note that on the way to accept his appointment at the port of Brest he stopped by the house of Ambroise Paré.

In 1797 Larrey was appointed Surgeon-in-Chief of the Napoleonic armies in Italy and later saw action during the French campaign in Egypt at the first Battle of Aboukir[44] on July 25, 1799. Respect and admiration for the doctor grew tremendously because of his battlefield activities. He didn't wait at the rear of the army for casualties. Instead, he flagrantly flung himself into the fray, ducking musket balls and shrapnel to treat the men where they fell. Apart from treating the wounds of French soldiers at this battle, he provided equal care to the injured Mamelukes, one of whom gave Larrey a talisman ring that he treasured and even wore at the Battle of Waterloo.

After the battle of Aboukir, Larrey's superiors criticized this impetuous behavior, but the wounded expressed genuine gratitude for the doctor's displays of courage. When the French troops were being evacuated, Larrey insisted that the wounded soldiers be repatriated first, and he personally organized their transportation to Toulon. Soon after this Larrey began to develop interest in treating the causes of scurvy, dysentery, and many other conditions that blighted Napoleon's troops in Egypt at the time. He also highlighted the importance of hygiene to the troops. Personal hygiene had never been a great priority for Napoleon. He once wrote to Josephine with the instruction, "Don't wash, my love, I will be home soon."

The war in Egypt revealed the surgeon's ability to supervise the care and the treatment of those wounded in action—a fact that didn't go unrecognized by Napoleon Bonaparte. When Dr. Larrey returned to Paris, he was appointed Chief Surgeon of the Consular Guard. At the beginning of the 18th century, Napoleon had openly stated his unambiguous views on military medicine, but his actions didn't always reflect

---

[44] The History of the French Revolution, Volume 5. By Adolphe Thiers.

his opinions. In 1800, he had a less than favorable idea about the French army medical service. "There is no medical service in the proper sense of the term,"[45] he said, and yet he apparently had high regard for Larrey.

Larrey's pioneering thesis on amputations in 1803 earned him wide recognition in the medical world. One year later, at the age of thirty-eight, he was officially appointed the "First Doctor" and received the esteemed *Legion d'honneur*, France's highest commendation, which was personally bestowed by first consul Napoleon Bonaparte who said, "Your work is one of the greatest conceptions of our age, it alone will suffice to ensure your reputation."

During the disastrous 1812 Russian campaign, Larrey was chief surgeon of the Grande Armée. The consummate organizer, he assembled all his surgeons in Berlin and gave them specific instructions to divide their staff into six "ambulance divisions." At the pivotal battles of Smolensk, Borodino, and the retreat from Moscow, he performed no less than two hundred amputations. The retreat became a real test of courage and tenacity for the Grande Armée. Lacking any serious logistical support and forced to endure withering Russian winter conditions, the retreat soon deteriorated into a rout.

Starved and exhausted, thousands of Napoleon's men succumbed to the elements while others experienced a serious breakdown of humanity and lost all semblance of civilization. One French sergeant wrote of an instance where an ambulance driver fell asleep, leaving the horse that pulled his ambulance unattended. During the night soldiers killed and ate the horse, rendering the ambulance surplus to requirements. Much to Larrey's chagrin, most ambulances had already exceeded their usefulness by this stage of the retreat. As the number of wounded and diseased men increased, there was little that could be done for them without access to the necessary supplies. Preferring not to remain in proximity to the sick and risk contracting their illnesses, ambulance drivers frequently ejected and abandoned their ailing cargo beside the road.

---

[45] Providing for the Casualties of War: The American Experience Through World. By Bernard D. Rostk (as quoted in Sieur, 1929). p. 855.

The soldiers who managed to reach the Berezina River and escape the marauding Cossacks were in a desultory state. Crossing the Berezina occurred between the twenty-sixth and twenty-ninth of November. Despite the incredibly brave exploits of the *pontonniers* (pontoon makers), whole battalions disappeared beneath the ice, never to surface again. Larrey wrote how he almost perished at the crossing. He made it over the bridge on two consecutive occasions to save his equipment and surgical instruments. During the third attempt to navigate the crowd of soldiers, one of them mentioned his name. Such was the respect and reverence for the doctor that, at this juncture, everyone on the bridge proffered assistance, and he was carried like a rock star during a crowd dive until he reached the end of the bridge and safety.

Despite having to deal with the horrendous conditions, Larrey and some of his staff continued attempting to perform their duties. Exhausted and suffering from typhoid, he arrived in Konigsberg on December 21, 1812. The hospitals of Konigsberg admitted about ten thousand of Napoleon's soldiers, but as they were admitted, the overworked staff at the hospital realized only a small number had been actually wounded. The majority were suffering from weather-related conditions such as frozen extremities. Physicians of that time referred to frostbite as a pest, a fever of congelation, which was terribly contagious. The heroic Larrey arrived at the hospitals to take care of the sick, but quickly succumbed to his illness. An old friend, Doctor Jacobi, gradually helped to restore his health.

The precise number of casualties incurred during the 1812 campaign will probably never be known, but it's estimated that Napoleon's Grand Armée began the invasion with around 673,000 men. Only 93,000 of them survived. Roughly 370,000 died of wounds and illness or exposure to the elements, and the Russians captured around 200,000.[46] Many of these prisoners also perished while others are reputed to have settled in Russia.

Such was his all-pervading influence on the French population at the time. Napoleon was able to raise three hundred thousand men within

---

[46] https://www.gutenberg.org/files/57185/57185-h/57185-h.htm.

three months of his return to Paris. In the ensuing battles, Larrey again displayed exceptional bravery on repeated occasions and was personally responsible for the evacuation of wounded French soldiers that were under attack by the dreaded Cossacks at the Heurtebise farm. Larrey remained fiercely loyal to his emperor and flatly refused to offer preferential treatment to the officers. He wrote: "General de Sparre was brought to my ambulance wounded. He demanded immediate attention, but, after examining his wound. I thought there were far more urgent cases to attend, so despite his protests, I made him wait his turn. I did the same with the Marshal Victor, Generals Grouchy and Cambronne, even though I regarded these men as my dear friends."[47]

When Napoleon was forced to abdicate at Fontainebleau, Larrey requested to be allowed to accompany the emperor into exile on the island of Elba. This request was vehemently refused because Napoleon wanted Larrey to remain with the soldiers of his beloved "Old Guard." Napoleon reciprocated Larrey's devotion by saying that "if the army ever erects a monument to express its gratitude, it should do so in honor of Larrey."

At Napoleon's final battle at Waterloo, Larrey received two sword cuts and was stabbed by a Prussian Ulhan's lance. Bleeding badly, he was captured and stripped almost naked by the Prussians, then brought before a General who demanded the doctor's immediate execution. The commander of the Prussian army (seventy-four-year-old Marshal Blücher) intervened on Larrey's behalf and spared his life on the premise that the doctor had saved the life of his son by caring for him on a battlefield a few years earlier. Larrey finally arrived back in Paris on September 15, 1815, and was warmly welcomed by his family in the city that was occupied by the victorious coalition.

After the restoration when many of Napoleon's men were tried as "Bonapartistes," the doctor remarkably retained his titles and function. Larrey luckily avoided imprisonment during the restoration of the French monarchy due to a highly complimentary report of his war services submitted by soldiers of all nationalities. On April 8, 1818, after twenty-eight

---

47 Napoleon and the marshals of 2nd Empire, two volumes complete in one (Philadelphia: j. b. Lippincott & co., 1855).

years of service and at the age of forty-nine, he ended his glorious career in the military.

Many historians claim that Larrey was an extremely vain, narcissistic man who frequently projected his vanity with malice. This description could have applied to most of Napoleon's Marshals, particularly that amazing cavalry officer Murat, who, according to Napoleon, "dressed like he was preparing to attend a carnival rather than a campaign," or words to that effect.

It is, however, undisputable is that Larrey's conduct during the Napoleonic Wars may have inspired the creation of the Red Cross and even the Geneva Convention. His name is engraved on the *Arc de Triomphe* in Paris, but it was ultimately his humane approach to caring for wounded regardless of allegiances or nationalities that remains as a guide to the behavior of doctors whenever they are compelled to decide between their duty to their patients and pressure from the authorities (in particular, the police or the army). Larrey wasn't the only reputable physician of the Napoleonic Wars.

CHAPTER EIGHT

In the 19th Century Navy

The British Royal Navy reserved the right to board American and other neutral merchant ships, even on the high seas. British ship captains also claimed many Americans—when they could ascertain who was actually American—because at that time there was nothing that could be identified as an American accent in the contemporary sense. Although certificates of citizenship were given to many American seamen in order to prevent them from being "press-ganged," it was relatively easy for British citizens to purchase or procure fake documents, both in America and in major British seaports. Hence, the Royal Navy treated them all with deep suspicion.

Back then the United States granted citizenship to almost all immigrants, but the British authorities claimed that nationality could not be renounced unless by permission of that nation. This implied that anyone born in the British Isles could not escape the obligation of serving in the navy simply by becoming a naturalized American citizen. On the basis of this, the Royal Navy arrogantly believed that it had the right to requisition anyone who spoke English. This inevitably resulted in literally thousands of Americans getting erroneously, or in many cases deliberately, press-ganged. It is estimated that from the start of the war with France in 1793 to the outbreak of war with America, between eight and ten thousand American seamen found themselves serving his mentally-challenged majesty King George III and serving in the British Royal Navy, but some actually volunteered. Some eminent historians claim that King George III was bi-polar, so this was possibly a case of British subjects getting "two for the price of one."

Life as a "Man o War" was relatively similar across the board, and many of those Americans who were press-ganged into serving with the British Royal Navy had to wait until after the War of 1812 before they would be repatriated. These unwilling matelots would have been attended by some of Admiral Lord Nelson's finest surgeons, who had the reputation as rough "sawbones" whose only skill was their ability to hack off limbs and pull teeth; however, they had discovered how to combat scurvy.

Sir William Dillon said of his surgeon, Thomas Grey, "Although an excellent scholar, being near-sighted with a defect in one of his eyes, we did not place much reliance on his ability at amputation."[48] The prospect of having a limb removed by a half-blind surgeon would not have inspired a lot of confidence from the patient. Thankfully this deficiency didn't apply to all of the naval surgeons, and at least some them had 20/20 vision, were well-educated, and were qualified in their field. Despite this the average death rate from amputation at the time was still around 33 percent.

To become a naval surgeon in the 18th and early 19th century, the candidate was required to serve a lengthy apprenticeship with a practicing surgeon ashore. Time could then be spent in a university or local hospital to learn the basics of anatomy, physiology, and pharmacology. Once they had acquired sufficient knowledge, they proceeded to the College of Surgeons in London for a rigorous examination. The Court of Examiners at the College of Surgeons would inform the navy at what level the newly qualified surgeon could serve on His Majesty's ships. Only the best were considered as competent enough to become a full-fledged ship's surgeon;

---

[48] The Seasick Admiral: Nelson and the Health of the Navy. By Kevin Brown (Pen and Sword, 2015).

most became a surgeon's mate, and these were denoted by their aptitude as first, second, or third class.

The college would specify the size of ship that the appointed surgeon could serve on and the kind of medical instruments that would be required for the task. With the onset of the Napoleonic Wars, Royal Navy surgeons were obliged to buy their own instruments and chest. A representative of the College of Surgeons would meticulously check these before allowing the surgeon to join the ship and assume the position.

The surgeon's quarters—the place where they practiced their profession—was usually located on the "Orlop deck" below the waterline. Despite being claustrophobic, dark, and oppressive, this was regarded as a comparatively safe area during a sea battle. The pungent rancid air emanating from the bilges wouldn't have helped much, either. Due to the low ceiling on the deck, the surgeon's gait would have been confined to a constant stoop. In the heat of battle, as thirty-two pounder guns boomed away directly above the surgeon's head, it was not necessarily the most placid working environment. Imagine attempting to remove an afflicted limb when the ship released a thunderous broadside or even worse, received one full on. When the ship wasn't actively engaged in naval or siege combat, the allocated sickbay would be situated in a partitioned area on a higher deck conducive to better light and air quality.

One of the most compelling accounts of naval warfare during the Napoleonic era can be found in the log written by Robert Young who served on board HMS Ardent. It's difficult to envisage the absolute cacophony and chaos that would have ensued when these timber framed leviathans received a broadside from all guns. Metal against wood was always a mismatch and while the surgeon, up to his ankles in warm blood, attempted to focus and perform his tasks, cannonballs would have been impacting in dangerously close proximity. Young relates the absolutely appalling conditions he endured during the Battle of Camperdown[49] on October 11, 1797: "I was employed in operating and dressing till near four in the morning, the action beginning about one in the afternoon. So

---

[49] Battle at Sea: 3000 years of naval warfare. By R.G. Grant (Dorling Kindersley Ltd.).

great was my fatigue that I began several amputations, under a dread of sinking before I should have secured the blood vessels. Ninety wounded were brought down during the action, the whole cockpit deck, cabins wing berths, and part of the cable tier, together with my platform, and my preparation for dressing were covered with them. So that for a time, they were laid on each other at the foot of the ladder."

A particularly debilitating illness that surgeons had to deal with during more sedentary times was venereal disease. The erstwhile remedies were a potential deterrent to curb the ardor of even the horniest matelots. The condition once established was usually treated by applying mercury to the afflicted parts and hoping for the best. Astringent injections of white vitriol (zinc sulfate) or barley water (administered under the prepuce or down the urethra) were also frequently prescribed. If your legs haven't crossed already, one surgeon suggested half an ounce of a concoction of Epsom salts and sugar of lead "to be injected down the yard (penis)." This would be followed by one dram of gum Arabic dissolved in three ounces of water if the scalding persisted, which it inevitably would. These treatments may not have cured the sailors' maladies but they would have definitely curbed their ardor for a while, if not permanently.

Seventeen-ninety-seven was a busy year for the British naval forces. In July 1797, Nelson was hit in the right arm by a musket ball shortly after stepping ashore leading a doomed assault on the Spanish island of Tenerife. Bleeding profusely, he was taken back to HMS Theseus where the injured limb was quickly amputated. On July 25 the ship's surgeon, James Farquhar,[50] wrote in his journal, "Compound fracture of the right arm by a musket ball passing thro a little above the elbow; an artery divided; the arm was immediately amputated." Some claimed that within thirty minutes of what must have been an unimaginably agonizing procedure, Nelson was up and about and yelling orders to his men. On the first of August, Farquhar noted: "Admiral Nelson; amputated arm; continued getting well very fast. Stump looked well; no bad symptoms whatever occurred."

---

[50] Making and Unmaking Disability: The Three-Body Approach. By Julie E. Maybee (Rowman & Littlefield).

A year later while commanding HMS Vanguard at the Battle of the Nile, Nelson received a musket ball in his head, fired by a French navy sniper, but still managed to secure a resounding victory against the French. The surgeon's log describes the treatment administered: "Wound on the forehead over the right eye, the cranium is bare for more than an inch, the wound three inches long. Discharged 1 September. The wound was perfectly healed on the first September but as the integuments were much enlarged, I applied (every night) a compress wet with a discutient embrocation for nearly a month which was of great service."[51]

In 1805 the surgeon Sir William Beatty tended Admiral Lord Horatio Nelson during his dying moments at the Battle of Trafalgar. The surgeon distinguished himself among the nineteen of one hundred and two casualties incurred during the action (including nine of the eleven amputees) that survived to tell the tale, though a few had developed certain speech impediments; however, the nature and cause of Nelson's mortal wounds were intentionally omitted from the naval journal of the Victory. Experts at the National Archives in Kew believe the omission was entirely deliberate because budding ambitious author Beatty wanted to save the details for publication in his own book that had the commercially viable title, *Authentic Narrative of the Death of Lord Nelson*, and was published in 1807. Smart move. In his book Beatty suggested that a division of a large branch of the left pulmonary artery was the cause of Lord Nelson's death. But what was the precise nature of Nelson's fatal wound? The French musket ball that did the damage struck Nelson on the left shoulder at the epaulette, with a force that first threw him onto his knees. It smashed two ribs and tore through his left lung, severing a major artery en route. Then having fractured the spine in the sixth and seventh vertebrae, damaging the spinal cord, it lodged five centimeters below his right shoulder blade in the muscles of his back. This corresponds with the angle and trajectory at which the ball was fired from the opposing French battleship.

Nelson stoically reported that he had difficulty breathing and felt a gush of blood inside his chest. Still conscious, he asked his valet to

---

[51] Nelson: The Sword of Albion. By John Sugden (Random House. 2014). p, 95.

turn him on to his right side, which gave him scant relief. Nevertheless, the Admiral remained conscious for a further three hours, but for most of that he would have suffered terrible agony. Beatty wrote, "the spinal injury by itself could have been mortal, but from it alone he could have survived 2-3 days although in miserable condition." Beatty eventually removed the ball aboard the Victory before arriving in England in December 1805. While extricating the offending projectile, he found "a portion of the gold-lace and pad of the epaulette, together with a small piece of his Lordship's coat firmly attached to it." Although Beatty's diagnosis and treatment were considered undisputable at the time, recent forensic neurosurgical analysis of Lord Nelson's fatal wound at Trafalgar reached a more thorough conclusion.

Blood loss from a torn pulmonary artery or from one of its branches and/or compression of vital structures by a hemothorax, was neither the only nor the main cause of his death, considering that the bleeding was just moderate and that modern ballistics excludes a major vessel in the trajectory of the musket ball. Lord Nelson, hot at first and cold thereafter, paralyzed, with back pain and a weak arterial pulse, died mostly of and in spinal shock, following complete damage of the mid-thoracic spinal cord. The cord was transected at T6-7 by the passage of a ball shot by a French musketeer, resulting in loss/paralysis of all neurological activity below the level of the lesion, including motor, sensory, reflex, and autonomic function. This prevented the body of the Admiral, despite its youth, from compensating for the chest bleed, contributing to end-organ cellular dysfunction/death from tissue hypoperfusion.[52]

The reason we refer to surgery being performed in the "operating theater" is because originally it was an actual theater, or rather amphitheater, where spectators paid for seats and waited to be entertained. Doctor Robert Liston, reputed to be the fastest operator of the day, elevated gross

---

52 Daniel E Nijensohn, "Admiral Horatio Lord Nelson's Death at the Battle of Trafalgar: A Neurosurgeon's Forensic Medical Analysis," Journal of Trauma & Treatment (June 5, 2017), https://www.hilarispublisher.com/open-access/admiral-horatio-lord-nelsons-death-at-the-battle-of-trafalgar-aneurosurgeons-forensic-medical-analysis-2167-1222-1000379.pdf.

incompetence to new heights. On one notable occasion he performed the only operation that sustained a 300 percent mortality rate. That must have taken some doing but Liston achieved it. Despite the fact that he could remove an extraneous limb in two and a half minutes, he managed to reduce that to twenty-eight seconds. His success rate during the formative years of his medical career was at best dubious, at worst horrendous. Whereas most surgeons at that time lost one in four patients, due to his speed and skill, Liston only lost about one in ten. On one particularly inauspicious occasion while he was performing a leg amputation, he brought down his knife with such speed that he removed his surgical assistant's fingers, along with the patient's leg. As he retracted the offending blade, it clipped a spectator's coattails, and he collapsed dead. The patient and Liston's assistant both died after their wounds became infected, and the spectator who collapsed was later discovered to have died of fright. On another occasion, in an effort to further increase his speed, he became a little over-animated and inadvertently chopped off the patient's testicles, as well as his leg. He eventually broke his personal record by completing an amputation in twenty five seconds.

He also once mistook a lump in a young boy's neck for a skin tag and removed it suddenly at the boy's home. It transpired that the offending lump turned out to be an aneurysm of the boy's carotid artery, which killed the poor lad stone dead. This is why Liston's surgery is the only one on record with a 300 percent mortality rate. His career was a catalogue of incompetence that would have deservedly embarrassed most of his contemporaries. Many years later, despite his downfalls, Liston pioneered the use of anesthetic and became a distinguished surgeon, but he had endured an ignominious reputation among those in the medical profession.

The surgeons at the battle of Waterloo accomplished wonders given the state of available medical science and the floods of men descending on them. One of their cruelest tasks, wrote William Gibney, "was to be obliged to tell a dying soldier who had served his king and country well on that day, that his case was hopeless, more especially when he was unable to realize the same for himself, and then to pass on to another, where skill might avail." It was a warm summer's day and the raging thirst afflicting the wounded men couldn't be satiated. Provisions were woefully inadequate and the little water to be found was tainted with human blood. William Gibney noticed, "The agony of some was so terrible, that they prayed to be killed outright than endure excruciating torture."

The end of the cataclysmic Napoleonic Wars in 1815, which culminated in the epic Battle of Waterloo, was for all intents and purposes the end of hostilities in Europe for almost 100 years, or so it is often stated. It actually wasn't because there were always empires to build and armies prepared to knock the living crap out of one another if one looked hard enough.

CHAPTER NINE

The Lady with the Limp

Anyone who has heard the name Florence Nightingale may also have heard the story of "The lady with the lamp," but how many know about the lady with the limp? International Nurses Day, celebrated almost everywhere throughout the world, occurs on Nightingale's birthday. A stark image has long been established in the public psyche of this feted feminist, this dedicated, incorruptible person who cared for British wounded in the Crimea. But dear Florence Nightingale was much more than a simple nurse. She was an assertive, complex, devious, ambitious woman whose modus operandi occasionally provoked more scorn than praise.

It was the age when the British Empire incorporated nearly one-fifth of the land surface of the globe, and these seemingly indomitable Victorians had harrumphed at nearly one quarter of the world's population. It was mighty indeed, if not a little despotic. "Mad Dogs and Englishmen" sweated profusely on the world's parade grounds in searing tropical heat under their heavy felt uniforms and thought that they were the masters of the universe. It was during this time of manic patriotism that a dubious alliance was formed between the British, the French, the

Ottomans, and the Sardinians against the Russians that culminated in what became known as the Crimean War.

Imagine for a moment, if you will, while the terrifying dissonance of battle still permeates the air, laying prostrate and wounded on a foreign field after catching a Russian bullet or Russian shrapnel. In the midst of all the blood, chaos, and mayhem you see a rather bumptious, garishly attired lady riding in your general direction at a steady, measured pace, accompanied by two heavily laden mules. She doesn't appear to be unduly worried, all things considered. Suddenly she releases a thunderous postern blast, unceremoniously dismounts her overladen mule and approaches you wearing a big, comforting smile. This adorable lady is the venerable Mrs. Mary Seacole and you're in luck, now you're in with a chance. Forget about the lady with the lamp and that abominable hospital in Scutari, you've got a chance to be saved by the lady with the limp. Mary's left foot was almost constantly swollen (possibly due to a dose of gout). As such, "lady with the limp" wouldn't have been an entirely inaccurate description.

Florence Nightingale may have scored a serious PR victory for her work in the Crimea, but she made little reference to one of the nurses who contributed greatly to the welfare of those same British troops. The sight of this gregarious, jolly woman arriving with her remedies was a mental and physical panacea for any wounded soldier on a foreign battlefield. In her lifetime Mary Seacole (1805–1881) achieved celebrity status and was even robustly acclaimed by the volatile Victorian age British public who, thanks to articles written by numerous journalists, were well-aware of her compassion, skill, and courage.

Many contemporary historians believe that Mary's contribution to the health and welfare of soldiers in the Crimea far exceeded those of Florence Nightingale. Once more the image may have exceeded the ability, and was on occasion painfully patronizing, but it couldn't detract from the good that this amazing woman did during her life.

Mary Seacole (or "Mother Seacole" as she affectionately became known to the troops) was born in Kingston, Jamaica, and christened Mary Jane Grant. Her father James Grant was a serving, hard-drinking

Scottish officer posted there as part of the British military contingent. Her hugely influential mother, also named Mary, was a creole (a person of mixed European and black descent) and a skillful exponent of traditional Jamaican herbal remedies and medicines. She ran "Blundell Hall," which was reputedly one of the finest hotels in Kingston, where she cared for invalid soldiers and their wives. This was the world that Mary Seacole was born into. Her education in medicine came mainly from her mother but benefited from other portentous influences. The authorities legally classified her as mulatto, a person who (like a creole) is born from of bi-racial parentage. Here the waters get a little muddy, though, because technically she was regarded as a quadroon, a person with one bi-racial parent and one white parent. Many years later Seacole wrote, "My father was a soldier, of an old Scotch family; and to him I often trace my affection for a camp-life, and my sympathy with what I have heard my friends call 'the pomp, pride, and circumstances of glorious war.'"[53]

As a soldier, James Grant's duty was to protect this lucrative British island against potential Spanish or foreign invasion. The island had belonged to Britain since May 10, 1655, when Admiral William Penn and General Robert Venables had forced Spain to relinquish possession and surrender. At the time of Seacole's birth, Jamaica was emerging as one of the many proverbial jewels in Victoria's empirical crown, as the world's leading exporter of sugar. Jamaica's Black population was known as the Maroons, and originally imported as slave labor from Africa by the British to work on the numerous sugar plantations. In 1800, just five years before Seacole was born, the island's three hundred thousand slaves outnumbered the white population by ten to one and the British authorities had been forced to contend with a few uprisings.

Some British soldiers ominously regarded a posting to the Caribbean early in the 19th century as a death sentence. This was mainly due to the various epidemics of yellow fever, cholera, malaria, and typhoid that occurred there. This reduced the effectiveness and numbers of British soldiers stationed there to such an extent that they were compelled to recruit

---

[53] Wonderful Adventures of Mrs Seacole in Many Lands. By Mary Seacole (Author) and Sara Salih (Editor, Introduction) (Penguin Classics, 2005).

former slaves. In 1807 the Mutiny Act was introduced, which granted freedom to all Black men who served in the British armed forces (who eventually received the same pay and rations as white soldiers). They were also supposed to be subjected to the same punishments, but the introduction of this law surreptitiously introduced a new form of inequality. Black soldiers joining the British West India regiments had to sign up for life, in contrast to their white counterparts who joined up for seven-year terms. It looked good on paper but in reality, there was still extensive racism among the ranks throughout the Victorian era and beyond.

Mary Grant married Englishman Edwin Horatio Hamilton Seacole on November 10, 1836, in Kingston, Jamaica. Edwin was a naval officer and reputed to be the illegitimate son of the hero of Trafalgar, 1st Viscount Horatio Nelson and his mistress Lady Hamilton. Mary Seacole's last will and testament contradicted this claim by stating that Edwin was not the illegitimate offspring but the godson of Nelson. He was the adopted son of Edwin Thomas Seacole, a local surgeon, apothecary, and male midwife, who raised the boy as his own.

Edwin never enjoyed a particularly healthy life and he died in 1844, which was coincidentally the same year that Seacole's mother also passed. Mary never remarried, preferring to dedicate her attention to managing her mother's hotel and eventual front-line nursing. She treated victims in the cholera epidemic of 1850 that claimed the lives of over thirty-two thousand Jamaicans. Her efficacious treatment of patients during this epidemic proved very beneficial in later years. She wrote, "I had gained a reputation as a skillful nurse and doctress, and my house was always full of invalid officers and their wives from Newcastle, or the adjacent Up-Park Camp. Sometimes I had a naval or military surgeon under my roof, from whom I never failed to glean instruction, given, when they learned my love for their profession, with a readiness and kindness I am never likely to forget."[54]

During her lifetime Seacole travelled extensively and on one occasion in 1852 she was travelling between Panama and the United States and

---

[54] Wonderful Adventures of Mrs Seacole in Many Lands. By Mary Seacole (Author) and Sara Salih (Editor, Introduction) (Penguin Classics, 2005).

spending time in the company of American traders. As she left the dinner table, she overheard an American say, "God bless the best yaller woman he ever made. If we could bleach her by any means, we would and make her acceptable in any company as she deserves to be." This infuriated Seacole, who mentioned in her autobiography, "I must say that I don't appreciate your friend's kind wishes with respect to my complexion. If it had been as dark as a nigger's, I should have been just as happy and useful, and as much respected by those whose respect I value: and as to his offer of bleaching me, I should, even if it were practicable, decline it without any thanks."[55]

She was reputed to have been a fiercely loyal patriot, and in her lifetime she made a number of journeys to the United Kingdom. Unfortunately, her loyalty and love for the country wasn't always reciprocated. It was during one of these visits that Seacole heard about the Crimean War. She was so moved by the distressing newspaper articles that she made applications to the War Office, British medical authorities, the army medical department, and the secretary of war to be allowed to go to the Crimea and tend to these desperately sick and wounded men. She was promptly refused and turned away at every juncture. Some claim that she even attempted to join Florence Nightingale's group of nurses. She didn't meet Nightingale at the time, but it's alleged that one of her chosen assistants refused to allow Mary to join the team. Nightingale's sister Parthenope unflatteringly described Florence as "a shocking nurse. She has little or none of what is called charity or philanthropy, she is ambitious, very, and would like to regenerate the world. I wish she could be brought to see that it is the intellectual part that interests her, not the manual. Florence's interests were in the administrative, at which she was very adept, however she could be impatient with other people and was reported especially to have not worked well with other women."[56] Consequently Parthenope,

---
[55] Wonderful Adventures of Mrs Seacole in Many Lands. By Mary Seacole (Author) and Sara Salih (Editor, Introduction) (Penguin Classics, 2005).
[56] Florence Nightingale: The Woman and Her Legend. By Mark Bostridge (Penguin, 2014).

81

whose name alone sounded like an intrusive surgical intervention, was never asked to provide a character reference for her sister. Meanwhile, deeply disappointed at the rejections, Mary observed, "Was it possible, that American prejudices against color had taken root here? Did these ladies shrink from accepting my aid because my blood flowed beneath a somewhat duskier skin than theirs?"[57]

No shrinking violet, Mary protested, pointing out that she had extensive experience, excellent references, and even knew some of the soldiers and regiments, having nursed them while they had been stationed in Jamaica. Her eventual value to the soldiers in the Crimea could to some extent be attributed to her extensive knowledge of the pathology of cholera, which she had contracted and recovered from. Undaunted, Mary made a further attempt to get to the Crimea when she applied for sponsorship and was flatly refused by the Crimean Fund, a charity founded by public subscription to support the wounded in Crimea. Despite all the adversity, she continued to explore ways to get to the war zone in the Crimea, where despite her detractors she was convinced that she would be able to do some good. It was quite serendipitous that Thomas Day, a relative of her deceased husband, was planning to go to the Crimea on business. After some discussion, she agreed to establish a limited company together with him that would become known as Seacole and Day.

January 27, 1855, was a momentous day when Seacole secured a passage to Constantinople (Istanbul) on board the Dutch ship Hollander that was making its maiden voyage. Armed with a letter of recommendation, she met and had a brief conversation with Florence Nightingale at the famous Scutari Army hospital in Turkey, which she refers to in her autobiography, "In half an hour's time I am admitted to Miss Nightingale's presence. A slight figure, in the nurses' dress; with a pale, gentle, and withal firm face, resting lightly in the palm of one white hand, while the other supports the elbow, a position which gives to her countenance a keen inquiring expression, which is rather marked. Standing thus in repose, and yet keenly observant, the greatest sign of impatience at any

---

[57] Idem

time a slight, perhaps unwitting motion of the firmly planted right foot was Florence Nightingale, that Englishwoman whose name shall never die, but sound like music on the lips of British men until the hour of doom. She has read Dr. F—'s letter, which lies on the table by her side, and asks, in her gentle but eminently practical and business-like way, 'What do you want, Mrs. Seacole – anything that we can do for you? If it lies in my power, I shall be very happy.'

"So I tell her of my dread of the night journey by cacique, and the improbability of my finding the 'Hollander' in the dark; and, with some diffidence, threw myself upon the hospitality of Scutari, offering to nurse the sick for the night. Now unfortunately, for many reasons, room even for one in Scutari Hospital was at that time no easy matter to find; but at last a bed was discovered to be unoccupied at the hospital washerwomen's quarters.

"My experience of washerwomen, all the world over, is the same, that they are kind soft-hearted folks. Possibly the soapsuds they almost live in find their way into their hearts and tempers, and soften them. This Scutari washerwoman is no exception to the rule, and welcomes me most heartily. With her, also, are some invalid nurses; and after they have gone to bed, we spend some hours of the night talking over our adventures, and giving one another scraps of our respective biographies. I hadn't long retired to my couch before I wished most heartily that we had continued our chat; for unbidden and most unwelcome companions took the washerwoman's place, and persisted not only in dividing my bed, but my plump person also. Upon my word, I believe the fleas are the only industrious creatures in all Turkey. Some of their relatives would seem to have migrated into Russia; for I found them in the Crimea equally prosperous and ubiquitous."[58]

Seacole stayed just one night at Scutari before taking another ship the following day across the Black Sea to the Crimean battle zone. When she arrived in the Crimea, she promptly set up at hotel Spring Hill, otherwise referred to as "Mrs. Seacole's hut" that was only a mile away from the

---

[58] Wonderful Adventures of Mrs Seacole in Many Lands. By Mary Seacole (Author) and Sara Salih (Editor, Introduction) (Penguin Classics, 2005).

British Army HQ. The first floor served as a restaurant while the second floor was requisitioned as a treatment area similar to a field hospital. She financed her operation by selling supplies while serving meals and copious amounts of alcohol. She then used her profits for the care of the ill and injured. Bear in mind that this woman was fifty years old at the time and quite portly, but despite her age and physical constitution, she maintained an irrepressible dynamism and endearing nature that acted like a virtual magnet to these soldiers far from home. It didn't take long for the name of Mother Seacole to spread through the entire British army. Higher officials referred to her condescendingly as a sutler, someone who follows the army and sells provisions to the troops, but she did more, much more, than just that.

Because she wasn't officially attached to any organization during the Crimean War, she had complete freedom of movement, which would have been denied to Florence Nightingale and her staff. In the Crimea, Seacole adopted a stringent routine treating those with medical conditions each morning, and then accompanied by two mules (one carrying medicaments and the other food and wine), she would travel to the front lines to treat casualties in situ. On a number of occasions, she tended wounded men from both sides while the battle was still raging.

William Howard Russell, special correspondent of *The Times*, wrote in 1856 of Mary Seacole, "In the hour of their illness, these men have found a kind and successful physician, who doctors and cures all manner of men with extraordinary success. She is always in attendance near the battlefield to aid the wounded and has earned many a poor fellow's blessing."[59] Whenever she approached the front lines, Mary Seacole's presence would have been immediately acknowledged because while defying bullets and cannonballs. She insisted on wearing highly conspicuous, brightly colored clothing.

Financially her Crimean venture left much to be desired because in 1857 she returned to London suffering from ill health and bankruptcy.

---

[59] Eyewitness Accounts Battles of The Crimean War. Paperback Eyewitness Accounts English. By William H. Russell.

Thanks to her outstanding service during the Crimean War, the British press rallied and advertised her pitiful plight. Many people donated to a fund for her, and even though Florence Nightingale was somewhat critical of Seacole's work, it was alleged that she secretly contributed to the fund. Later that year and at the insistence of those close to her, she decided to write an autobiography titled (somewhat ostentatiously) *Wonderful Adventures of Mrs. Seacole in many lands.*[60] Unlike most budding authors, her fame was such at the time that she had no problem finding a publisher to print these memoirs. The ensuing book sold remarkably well and she lived out her remaining years in relative comfort. Mary Seacole died quietly as a direct result of a cerebral hemorrhage in London May 14, 1881, and was sadly soon forgotten.

Since 1981 on the anniversary of her death, there's a wreath-laying ceremony held at her grave each year, and in 2005 Penguin Classics reprinted her book. The two hundredth anniversary of Seacole's birth was celebrated with the unveiling of a lost painting of her at the National Portrait Gallery in London. A fundraising campaign in her name raised over half a million pounds and led to the unveiling of a beautiful statue of Mary Seacole on the grounds of St. Thomas' hospital, London. This memorial statue is believed to be the U.K.'s first in honor of a black woman. Her methods of treatment may have been regarded as unorthodox by the Victorian medical establishment, and many claimed that she profited from the British army, but she rightfully earned her place as one of the famous nurses in history. Mary's memory lives on. God bless her.

---

[60] Wonderful Adventures of Mrs Seacole in Many Lands. By Mary Seacole (Courier Dover Publications, 2019).

CHAPTER TEN

African American Slave Medicine

One of the most ignominious and disturbing aspects of American medical history relates to the intrinsically evil slave trade, which occurred during the Antebellum (approximately 1820–1860). This was a notorious period in the history of the Southern United States that began during the late 18th century and continued until the onset of the American Civil War in 1861. Men, women, and children forcibly taken from their native lands were transported across the Atlantic Ocean to the Americas during the 18th and 19th centuries in the most dehumanizing, claustrophobic conditions imaginable. They were regarded as the lowest form of human life by most of their owners, but a healthy slave was a valuable one, so their health depended primarily on the benevolence and generosity of their owners. The ubiquitous practice of miscegenation, although illegal, was largely condoned and practiced by many slave owners that sincerely believed in the superiority of the White race popularized by the antebellum south.

Most of these African slaves retained their own native medical practices and knowledge. Their botanical healing recipes were often relatively complex and required considerable time and effort to prepare. One recipe for dysentery required boiling a "teacup of logwood chips in a pint of sweet milk," then boiling another ten minutes with sugar, and finally burning "four tablespoons of brandy"[61] in a plate, then stirring it into the milk mixture. On the whole slave remedies tended to be more simplistic than white medicines. Teas or poultices were usually made combining the ingredients of one or two plants. One particular herbal cure used by African American slaves was derived from the asafetida plant. Asafetida is a perennial relative of silphium of Cyrene and has characteristics of plants in the fennel family. Native to India and Iran, it is still widely used in Indian cuisine, and was probably imported by European settlers. As its name suggests, asafetida has a fetid, almost putrid odor to it, hence it is commonly referred to as stinking gum, or Devil's dung. The Silphium plant was used in classical antiquity as a seasoning, perfume, aphrodisiac, and medicine. Ancient Greeks and Romans also used this plant as a contraceptive.

When the slaves couldn't procure indigenous ingredients, they used what they considered to be equivalents such as snakeroot, may apple, red pepper, boneset, pine needles, comfrey, and red oak bark, among many others. Slave healers understood the various preparations of pokeweed and how to extract its curative properties. Sassafras root tea was a particularly popular seasonal blood cleanser. Jimsonweed was intended as a cure for rheumatism, chestnut leaf tea for asthma, and mint and cow manure tea for chest infections and tuberculosis (via consumption).

West African slaves introduced herbal knowledge to their respective communities and also surreptitiously imported the actual seeds. This was achieved by two means: first by using necklaces made from wild licorice seeds, which were worn initially as a protective amulet. Second, the despicable holds below the decks of the ships were lined with straw that in some cases contained the seeds of African grasses and other plants. Some of these were planted over in the New World's fertile earth. Many slaves discovered that the West African climate is similar to that of southern American states, which may have been conducive to the cultivation of

---

[61] The John Couper Family at Cannon's Point. By T. Reed Ferguson (Mercer University Press, 1994).

the seeds they brought. When this wasn't possible, they found and utilized equivalents to their own plant species. Native Americans as well as White Europeans used some of the herbal remedies disseminated by captive Africans.

One of the most pervasive practices involved Slave midwives at a time when infant mortality among their communities was at least 30 to 35 percent. The living standards of slave children born into depravity were exceedingly poor. It is estimated that newborns weighed on average less than twenty-three kilos. Many of the maladies encountered by the slaves were a direct result of poor nutritional practices and disease. The punitive work they were forced to endure during pregnancy and postnatal practices, and possibly genetic factors, all contributed to poor health.

Slave midwives would have been aware of certain herbs used to treat "female complaints" and to ease childbirth. Slaves preferred their own doctors to white doctors, and their adherence to the widely prescribed humors, purging, and bloodletting. Some contemporary medical specializations, such as obstetrics and gynecology, still owe a great debt to enslaved women who became, in many cases, unwitting experimental subjects.

The plantation owner regarded the health of his slaves as critical to the economic welfare of the community. Failure to report slave illnesses to a farm's overseer or owner could result in severe punishment. In many cases the mistress of the plantation was charged with the responsibility of the health of slaves, which must have put a strain on the marriage, among other things. But these were not the demure Scarlett O'Hara types of *Gone with the Wind*. These mistresses knew full well that suitable nutrition and clean clothing were essential to maintain the health of the slave work force. Their productivity and health depended on these aspects. When a serious illness was detected, patients were sometimes moved from the slave quarters to the "sick house" where they would receive medical care.

In the Old South during the antebellum, large families were relatively common. The mistresses were often relegated to being mobile baby factories, but news of pregnancy and imminent birth was rarely regarded as a joyous occasion because frequent births took a toll on women's health.

Childbirth was a source of great anxiety and fear because there was always the omnipresent possibility that death could occur during labor, and this was a cause for serious concern for the mistress and her husband. The complications that could arise from a difficult birth, which could take hours or even days, included prolapse of the uterus, clearing the body of the afterbirth, puerperal (a deadly infection of the uterus), and the inability to breastfeed the child.

When the white mother encountered complications after childbirth, slave women were occasionally requisitioned to be wet nurses for white infants.

In 1858 Savannah Medical College professor Juriah Harriss published an article in a medical journal[62] stating that the ability to accurately determine the market value of "Black bodies" was one of the key professional competencies required by southern doctors. Insurance companies often hired White doctors to examine enslaved men and women before issuing life insurance policies to protect slaveholders' financial well-being. Most of these doctors were kept on an annual retainer to help ensure the health and well-being of the slaves.

Freed African American former slave Thomas Foote[63] recalled the experiences of his free mother, a respected healer known as the "doctor woman." As a young woman she worked for a certain Dr. Ensor, whom Foote described as a well-known homeopathic doctor. Foote's mother prescribed medicine compiled from the same leaves, herbs, and roots that Dr. Ensor used. The white community didn't trust the "doctor woman," but the slaves openly confided in her even though the masters were not exempt from personally administering medical care. (Quite a number of the plantation owners were qualified physicians.) The main problem of the masters came as a result of their attempts to coerce African American women slaves to use the services of a physician because they preferred

---

[62] The Richmond Medical Journal, Volume 1. MD. By E.S Gaillard and W.S. McChesney (1866).

[63] "Thomas Foote, Cockeysville, Maryland." Federal Writers' Project: Slave Narrative Project, Vol. 8, Maryland, Brooks-Williams (1936). https://www. loc.gov/resource/mesn.080/?sp=17&st=text.

their indigenous botanical remedies. This could foster other complications because it wasn't unusual for contagious illnesses to spread to other occupants on the plantation and surrounding areas.

When Congress forbade the continued importation of slaves to the United States in 1808, the slave owners relied heavily on physicians to establish a natural increase of the current slave population through selective breeding. This law coincided with the expansion of labor-intensive cotton crop farming in the lower south and west. From this point on black women were evaluated on the basis of their capacity to be good "breeders" for their owners, as well as hard productive workers. Insidious white southern doctors capitalized on their unfettered access to enslaved African American women to enhance their own frequently sordid reputations. The physicians had carte blanche from the slave owners to conduct some horrific experiments on slave women's bodies in a vain attempt to produce medical and surgical developments. The main problem was that innumerable slave women succumbed or were permanently maimed as they submitted to the scalpel administered with the consent of their owners.

Physicians were allowed to conduct experimental surgeries without anesthesia, even when they admitted that they were unlikely to cure the patient or save her life. One of the leading exponents of experimental surgery and women's reproductive health was James Marion Sims[64] who is often credited as the "father of modern gynecology." There are statues to this man in many American cities. His research was frequently conducted on African American women slaves without anesthesia and without their consent. Because of his involvement in this insidious practice, many medical ethicists, historians, and others have called for those monuments to be removed, destroyed, and ground to dust. Sims has many detractors and rightfully so, but there are also those who claim that he was a pioneer, an innovator. Can the same be said of Josef Mengele? He also practiced on unwilling subjects.

---

[64] Clinical notes on uterine surgery. By James Marion (William Wood & Co. 1971).

Among other things Sims established a surgical technique to repair vesicovaginal fistula, a ubiquitous 19th century complication resulting from childbirth, in which a tear between the uterus and bladder would cause incessant, agonizing pain and urine leakage. It's hardly surprising that these poor unfortunate souls preferred their own remedies. The close quarter interaction between African Americans and whites functioned on many levels. Medical knowledge would have been frequently exchanged due to the fact that many slave children were playmates, willing or otherwise, of white children. Moreover, African American slave women were often requisitioned to nurture the plantation owners' children. This would have established emotional and cultural bonds, but it was always at the behest of the master. The bonds were in most cases guided by economic considerations rather than philanthropic ones.

CHAPTER ELEVEN

Blue + Gray = Red.

Disease consumed twice as many lives in the American Civil War than combat related deaths. In this bitterly contested conflict that divided a young nation, approximately one in ten Union soldiers were killed or incapacitated, and the reapers' tally was a high as one in four on the Confederate side.

The criteria for enlistment on both sides were somewhat lax to say the least. According to the 1861 US Sanitary Commission Report, three quarters of the soldiers discharged from the Union Army should never have even been allowed to enlist on medical grounds. Army Regulation 1297 stipulated the regulations for physical exams pertaining to enrolment: "In passing a recruit the medical officer is to examine him stripped; to see that he has free use of all his limbs; that his chest is ample; that his hearing, vision and speech are perfect; that he has no tumors, or ulcerated or extensively cicatrized legs; no rupture or chronic cutaneous affection; that he has not received any contusion, or wound of the head, that may impair his faculties; that he is not a drunkard; is not subject to convulsions; and has no infectious disorder; nor any other that may unfit him for military service.

Consequently, during that first terrible year almost one-third of the Union Army reported sick, and alcohol was widely abused in both Union and Confederate armies during the Civil War. One Union General was perplexed by the behavior of his soldiers. Every night a picket guard was sent to an outpost one and a half miles from Fort Monroe, Virginia. They returned to the post the following morning and caused trouble due to being inebriated. Thorough investigations failed to determine the source of their whiskey. Searches of canteens and equipment revealed nothing suspicious. There was, however, something peculiar about the way that the men dispatched for guard duty always held their muskets vertically. The mystery was solved when their muskets were examined. Every barrel of these weapons was filled to the brim with whiskey, too much of which could be seriously detrimental to health.

Whiskey distilled with questionable methods carried with it the threat of poisoning the drinker. The moonshiners might use clear alcohol as a base then add water to the mixture and chewing tobacco to simulate the color and flavor of the real thing (possibly destroying the taste buds in the process). Harsher ingredients occasionally provided that "clout" drinkers expected from their whiskey. An 1860 inspection of liquor samples in Cincinnati discovered ersatz whiskey containing sulfuric acid, red pepper, caustic, soda, potassium, and strychnine. It was no wonder that it became widely referred to by the troops as "rotgut." In fact, a plethora of colorful nicknames were attributed to alcohol distributed during the Civil War, such as "Oh be joyful," "Blue ruin," and "Forty Rod." Alcohol of varying potency and toxicity was widely used and abused by both Union and Confederate armies.

Most of the women abstained from indulging the devil alcohol during the Civil War. Both sides employed more than 20,000 women in military hospitals and around half this number served as nurses. This chapter will cover the contributions made by some illustrious names such as Mary Bickerdyke, Clara Barton, Dorothea Dix, Louis May Alcott, and Tillie Pierce. They all hailed from diverse backgrounds. Dorothea Dix made it her personal métier to recruit only middle class, white women between the ages of thirty-five and fifty who resided in the Washington, D.C.

area. In Indiana and other states, Ladies Aid Societies also made a point of recruiting only local women. African American women living on both sides, enslaved and free, performed various duties including nursing, and it's estimated that around 11 percent of women medical workers were of African American descent.

Augusta Jane Evans, Juliet Opie Hopkins, Kate Cummings, and Sally Louisa Tompkins were among some of the notable nurses that contributed to the Confederate cause. But they were not called nurses—that title was reserved for men. These tenacious, hard-working, dedicated southern belles were politely referred to as "Matrons" (among other things, depending on the severity of the wound). Although many of these ladies subscribed to diametrically opposed ideologies, they all had certain things in common: courage, compassion, and dedication to the care of wounded and dying men.

It was a war that commenced with only one hundred doctors and culminated with over 13,000 doctors serving in the Union Army Medical Corp alone. The doctors who acquired their positions in the army could only be appointed by a designated commission or by the president or state governor. But even back then it could have been a question of whom you know rather than what you know.

One particular powerful presence during the Civil War was Mary Ann Ball Bickerdyke (1817–1901), a Civil War nurse who became an active agent for the United States Sanitary Commission. The Union soldiers, who greatly valued the care and attention she selflessly lavished on them affectionately referred her to as "Mother Bickerdyke," but she had a run of bad luck during her early years. Some speculated that an albatross rather than a stork had brought her.

Mary Ann was born in in 1817 in Knox County, Ohio. After her mother's death her father, Hiram Ball (a farmer), sent his seventeen-month-old daughter away to be raised by her grandparents. When they died, Mary Ann went to live with her Uncle Henry Rodgers in Oberlin, Ohio. At the tender age of sixteen, she studied briefly with a doctor of botanic medicine, learning the healing qualities of herbs and fruits, and the health benefits of fresh air and cleanliness. After being moved around more times than a chess piece, she met and married Robert Bickerdyke, a widower with three children, on April 27, 1847. In 1856 they all settled in Galesburg, Illinois, and by all accounts it was a happy marriage. A few years later Robert died in 1858 at the age of fifty-four.

Moreover, infant mortality was ubiquitous back then. Their third child, Martha, died at the age of two just a year after Robert's passing. Mary Ann, now a bereaved widow, needed to find some way of supporting her sons Hiram and James and her three stepchildren. In May 1861, now forty-four-year-old Mary Ann attended services at the Brick Congregational Church in Galesburg and heard the pastor read a moving letter from Benjamin Woodward, a Galesburg physician and regimental surgeon for the 22nd Illinois infantry requesting medical volunteers. Although Mary hadn't really experienced any extensive formal education, she decided to employ her scant knowledge of herbicidal remedies to provide what care she could for sick and wounded soldiers.

After the good townsfolk of Galesburg vowed to care for her children, Mary Ann had free reign to supervise and deliver supplies to the medical facility at Cairo in Illinois. When she arrived there, she was appalled by the horrific conditions she witnessed. With the help of a young soldier named Andy Somerville, she rampaged through camp like a hurricane, cleaning and disinfecting tents, establishing field kitchens, and introducing badly needed army laundries. She also provided fresh straw and clean water for the sick and wounded men previously housed in squalid, vermin infested tents and had wooden barrels cut in half so they could bathe and dress in clean clothes provided by the congregation in Galesburg.

Mary Ann was also responsible for setting up boiling kettles over campfires that she used to cook hot soup, porridge, tea and coffee, and even baked bread in ad hoc brick ovens. Using her agricultural background, she bought and bartered for eggs, milk, and fresh vegetables from the local farmers, which she used to prepare nutritious meals in field kitchens.

After completely reorganizing the camp at Cairo, Mary Ann felt that she had the obligation to remain in service. There was still work to do. She was required to maintain standards in Cairo, as well as at other camps and hospitals where desultory conditions existed. Thus began years of military service, improving sanitation and living conditions while nursing the countless afflicted Union and Confederate soldiers.

Mary Ann became instantly popular with the men. She was a matronly woman with a friendly face, wearing her gray calico dress and shaker bonnet she waltzed among the soldiers offering comforting words and considerate smiles as she personally doted over each soldier, many of whom regarded her as the mother they so badly missed. In November of 1862, she went on a fundraising tour for the Sanitary Commission and visited several towns relating stories of her traumatic experiences in the war. Her lectures were resoundingly popular and the audiences donated generously to this cause. When one faithful assistant affectionately named her "Mother," the name stuck, and she became known to both generals and soldiers alike as Mother Bickerdyke, which rightfully sealed her place in history.

The duties of Southern nurses were usually confined to providing religious counsel, aiding the mortally wounded soldier face a "good death," and writing letters to the family about the passing of a loved one. Their duties depended largely on whether the matron was serving in a Confederate hospital facility or operating in the field where the work was considerably more diverse and frequently more labor-intensive.

As most Southern states declared their independence and seceded from the Union into the Confederate States of America, Augusta Jane Evans a nationally renowned novelist and the eldest daughter of a family of eight children evolved to become a fervent Southern patriot. She wholeheartedly supported the Confederacy in every feasible way she could. This entailed volunteering her services at a hospital, singing patriotic songs to rally the Confederate troops and organizing the women of her hometown Mobile Alabama to do necessary war work. Mobile wasn't a particularly large city at the time, but it was important to the despicable slave trade. One of the reasons that she so enthusiastically supported the southern cause was because her brothers had joined the 3rd Alabama Regiment. On one occasion when she traveled to visit them in Virginia Union soldiers from Fort Monroe fired directly at her small group. She wrote to a friend, "O! I longed for a Secession flag to shake defiantly in their teeth at every fire! And my fingers fairly itched to touch off a red-hot-ball in answer to their chivalric civilities." She set up a private hospital in Mobile, and soldiers stationed in proximity called their camp "Camp Beulah" in honor of Augusta's novel. It was later reported that her book *Macaria*, also known as *Altars of Sacrifice* (1864), had such detrimental effect on the morale of Union soldiers that some officers ordered copies of it to be burned. She survived the war and died May 9, 1909. Her mortal remains were buried in Mobile Alabama.

Another notable Confederate supporter and nurse was Juliet Opie Hopkins. She was born on a plantation in Jefferson County, Virginia (present-day West Virginia). After her marriage to Chief Justice Arthur F. Hopkins of Mobile, Alabama, she relocated there. When the War began, she was forty-five years old, affluent, and already the mother of several children. She followed the Alabama troops to Virginia. During the Civil War, while working at a supply depot in Richmond over a four-month period from December 1861 until April 1862, she personally oversaw and arranged the conversion of three tobacco factories into hospitals. One of these facilities was collectively large enough to house over 500 patients, which she visited on a daily basis. Her personal contributions were along the same lines as Augusta, handling patient correspondence and supplying reading materials for the soldiers.

When a wounded soldier died, Juliet would personally send a lock of their hair to their next of kin. But she didn't confine her activities to these hospitals. During the Battle of Seven Pines on May 31, 1862, she sustained two serious hip wounds at that left her with a permanent limp. It would take more than a century before she would be awarded the Confederate Medal of Honor for this action. The Confederate troops gave her the nickname "Florence Nightingale." In 1862 Confederacy merged the patient load at the smaller hospitals into the larger facilities at other locations throughout Alabama. During the course of the War, she and her husband donated more than $200,000 to the support of this hospital and other similar agencies. Juliet died August 3, 1890, and was buried at Arlington.

One of the most cataclysmic battles fought during the American Civil War occurred at a small Pennsylvanian town called Gettysburg. This clash of giants, contesting ideologies that dealt out death in a gargantuan three-day struggle to claim the field remains emblazoned in the minds of everyone who is familiar with the name. There have been numerous expertly written accounts detailing the battle, and there's very little that one can add to that. The raw emotive sentiments and folk myths surrounding this battle still occasionally contradict the abundant, de facto academic assessments of military historians. This second great rebel invasion of Union soil north of the Potomac culminated in a battle that would ultimately contribute to deciding the uncertain future of a young nation. It was one battle in a contentious, destructive four-year war that claimed the lives of over six hundred thousand. Some say that Gettysburg was America's Waterloo, and there are indeed similarities apart from the distinction that Waterloo was a Pan-European affair while this was an entirely American engagement.

It is indeed difficult to add anything to what historians through the decades have meticulously dissected and studied Gettysburg from every conceivable perspective. They have proposed educated opinions on the strategy, tactics, and mindsets of the key incumbents to the point of saturation. Despite all that interest in the battle, the name of Gettysburg continues to resonate down through the decades, inspiring new perceptions, new analysis, and new stories. This chapter won't focus on the semantics and intricacies of the actual battle for obvious reasons, but it will relay some of the devastating experiences of some of the young angels inadvertently swept up in the sequence of events and confronted with the grim reality of battle casualties.

Those armchair generals and wonderful reenactors all harbor their own theories on how victory or defeat was achieved, and at the drop of a hat they're usually all too willing to offer their opinions. Very few mention the medical services, or more specifically the experiences of one young fifteen-year-old girl who was there, who witnessed the intolerable suffering of the wounded as they lay bleeding out and dying on the cold stone floor of a nearby farm in close proximity to the battlefield.

This is the often-neglected human aspect that weighs just as heavily as the magnanimous decisions of generals and officers. The names and places they describe have long since become ingrained, iconic in American military history, but seen through the innocent frightened eyes of one particular young girl they have different connotations. Matilda "Tillie" Jane Pierce brings these places to life again and tells how the events affect her life and her perspective. Tillie didn't volunteer to be a nurse; she wasn't coerced, either. She was just in the wrong place at the wrong time, but that didn't prevent her from stepping up to the plate when she had to. She was the daughter of James and Margaret Pierce, born on March 11, 1848, in Gettysburg, where she resided in 1860 with her parents, elder brothers, and elder sister, namely James Shaw, William H., and Margaret.

Father James Pierce was a butcher who lived and worked on the southwest corner of south Baltimore and Breckenridge streets. The Pierce family residence is still there. When war broke out the Pierce brothers enlisted in the Union army, James Jr. as a private with the 1st Regiment Pennsylvania Reserves, Company K, and William as a private with the 15th Pennsylvania Cavalry, Company E. James' company was the only one in the Army of the Potomac composed entirely of Gettysburg-Adams County men who had heeded the call to arms delivered by Gov. Andrew Curtin in June 1863.[65]

The civilians of Gettysburg formed a militia that became known as the 26th Pennsylvania Emergency Militia. Tillie wrote that the 26th Pennsylvania was "armed to the teeth." She saw her father James Pierce drilling with Company G of the militia on the fields just outside of town. Before long the 26th Pennsylvania would be called upon to defend the civilians of Gettysburg.

---

[65] (Authors note: I discovered this particular story during a visit to Gettysburg with my wife one week before the 150th Anniversary. After strolling around the battlefield with an expert guide, we visited a delightful couple at a place called the Wiekert farm. They told me about this truly amazing young lady and I told them that if I ever write about battlefield nurses. I will definitely include her name and her exploits.)

When men from Maj. Gen. Jubal A. Early's Confederate command of the Army of Northern Virginia began to encroach the outskirts of Gettysburg on June 26, they encountered little resistance from the militia that has assembled at the town's perimeter. It only took one volley from the Confederates to send them scampering for cover. That same afternoon Tillie, who was a student attending Rebecca Eyster's Young Ladies Seminary located on High Street, was taking a test when a boy arrived yelling, "The Rebels are on the outskirts of town!" All the students and Mrs. Eyster rushed to the front porch and looked north in the direction of the Lutheran Theological Seminary where they noticed "a dense mass moving toward town." Mrs. Eyster wasted no time in immediately sending the girls home.

After arriving home Tillie saw men on horseback followed by infantry. She wrote, "What a horrible sight! There they were human beings clad almost in rags, covered with dust, riding wildly, pell-mell down the hill toward our home shouting, yelling most unearthly, cursing, brandishing their revolvers, and firing left and right."

During its temporary occupation of the town, the Confederate force pillaged everything they could lay their hands on. General Early had demanded 1,000 pairs of shoes and 500 hats or, as an alternative, $10,000 in cash. But when the town officials pleaded poverty, Early ordered his men to run riot. They only requisitioned a few horses, one of which was owned by the Pierce family. Tillie's father pleaded with looting Confederates for the return of his horse, but they were not really in a listening mood.

When one of Tillie's neighbors named Henrietta Schriver said she was taking her two children to a potentially safer location at her father Jacob Weikert's house out on the Taneytown Road, just south of Gettysburg, Tillie's parents asked Henrietta if their daughter could join them.

At around 1:00 p.m., Tillie, along with Mrs. Schriver and the two Schriver children, began to head south toward the Weikert house. Tillie recalled seeing the fierce battle erupting on Seminary Ridge. After a short but arduous journey, the women reached their destination safely. Some time later, a Union artillery passed nearby and a caisson exploded in front of the house. A soldier wounded by the blast was picked up and brought to the Weikert home. Tillie noticed that "his eyes were blown out of their sockets and that he seemed to be one black mass, so severely had he been burned by the explosion." After the artillery had passed, infantry began passing the Weikert house. Tillie noticed that the men in the ranks appeared to be thirsty, so she got a wooden bucket and "carried water to them until the spring was drained."

That afternoon wounded Union soldiers began drifting back to the Weikert farm, which was soon transformed into a field hospital. That evening Tillie and Beckie Weikert, Jacob Weikert's daughter, went out to the barn. Tillie described the shock of seeing that impromptu field hospital for the first time: "Nothing before in my experience had ever paralleled the sight we then and there beheld. There were the groaning and crying, the struggling and dying, crowded side by side, while attendants sought to aid and relieve them as best they could. We were so overcome by the sad and awful spectacle that we hastened back to the house weeping bitterly."

Exhausted by the day's tumultuous events Tillie slept soundly that night. At ten o'clock in the morning of July second, she noticed more infantry passing and again began to offer water to them. She saw a disheveled soldier crawling along on his hands and knees. A Union officer approached the afflicted man and began severely berating him while demanding that he get to his feet. When the soldier didn't respond the officer struck him several times with the flat of his sword. The now-wounded soldier was brought into the house where the nurses tended him and a few hours later he recovered.

By mid-afternoon she distinctly heard the ominous roar of cannon fire coming from an area behind the house as the assault on Little Round Top commenced. Tillie saw her brother's regiment, along with the rest of the brigade assuming positions on a hillside in proximity to the Jacob Weikert barn. The brigade advanced down the hill and delivered a volley toward Brig. Gen. Joseph B. Kershaw's Confederate troops. After repulsing the Confederates back beyond a stone wall, the Union brigade halted and held that position until the evening of July third.

She later wrote: "Amputating benches had been placed about the house. I must have become inured to seeing the terrors of battle; else I could hardly have gazed upon the scenes now presented. I was looking out of one of the windows facing the front yard. Near the basement door, and directly underneath the window I was at, stood one of these benches. I saw them lifting the poor men upon it, then the surgeons sawing and cutting off arms and legs, then again probing and picking bullets from the flesh.... To the south of the house and just outside of the yard, I noticed a pile of limbs higher than the fence."[66]

Tillie described seeing every room packed tight with casualties in all stages of suffering. The floors would have been steeped inches deep with congealed blood, and the air would have been rendered foul with putrid odors. All accompanied by a deathly, resonant chorus of tormented moans, cries and screams of pain. No place for a fifteen-year-old girl under normal circumstances. Thankfully social media didn't encumber her or nothing would have gotten done. She survived her experiences and later wrote extensively about them.

She would eventually be reunited with her family, who miraculously all survived the ordeal unscathed. Tillie hadn't had much sleep the past few days, which made her understandably cranky. She had walked the battlefield, seen the carnage and witnessed some terrible things. She would carry the memory of that battle in her heart for the rest of her natural life. Her diary is a heart-rending testament to courage, tenacity, and suffering that echoes to this day. Tillie married her long-time sweetheart lawyer Horace T. Alleman in 1871. They had three children and lived in Selinsgrove, Pennsylvania. In her later years she became a prominent member of the Women's Relief Corps of Selinsgrove. She died March 15, 1914, of cancer after spending five months in the University of Pennsylvania Hospital Philadelphia.[67] This story would not have been possible without the wonderful assistance provided by Beth and

---

[66] At Gettysburg, or, What a Girl Saw and Heard of the Battle. By Matilda "Tillie" Pierce Alleman.

[67] Idem

Gerry Hoffman, the current owners of the Wiekert farm, Gettysburg, Pennsylvania.

American authorities were not prepared for war, and at the outbreak of the American Civil War the U.S. Sanitary Commission faced some serious challenges. It provided the Union Army with medical supplies and equipment purchased from donations, but had no official authority to enforce its advice or to compel the use of its supplies and equipment. It did, however, play an important part in shaping the medical care Union soldiers received. The inadequacy of the Medical Department to provide sufficient triage and medical assistance to battle casualties during the first year of the war was accentuated by the disaster at the first major battle of the war fought at Bull Run in Manassas, Virginia, July 21, 1861. It illustrated how woefully unprepared the Union Army was from a medical standpoint. Fortunately, at Bull Run, casualty figures were relatively small compared with future battles (North, 481 killed, 1011 wounded; South, 387 killed, 1582 wounded).

During the American Civil War, author of *Little Women* Louisa May Alcott, rested her quill and worked for a short time in one of these facilities as a nurse. L. M. Alcott had no formal training, but on December 11, 1862, she went to the Union hospital in Georgetown, outside of Washington, D.C., to volunteer her services. She would later relate her experiences in her book *Hospital Sketches* (1863), which tells the story of a bedside army nurse.[68]

She endured about six weeks, but that was long enough to provide her with inspiration and vital information for some of her future literary works. The real credit for any involvement in the war should be more attributed to her family rather than to the author herself. The Alcott family maintained a strongly humanitarian stance throughout this turbulent period in American history by providing a "safe house" for the revered Underground Railroad that assisted former slaves in their attempts to reach safety in the north.

---

[68] Hospital Sketches. By Louisa May Alcott.

The technology of warfare had created devastating weapons capable of inflicting horrific injuries, but sadly advances in medical science still lagged way behind. Moreover, by the time of the American Civil War, surgeons had not kept pace.

Surgeons and nurses at that time had scant knowledge of bacterial infections, therefore many of the surgical procedures were performed without even the most rudimentary preparations, such as using soap and water or disinfectant. The place was a humid, rancid-smelling hovel, inadequately supplied, overcrowded, chaotic, and completely unsanitary. Preventable diseases such as typhoid and dysentery were rampant due to poor knowledge of epidemiology. Civil War army nursing was not for the fainthearted or reticent, therefore Nurse Alcott would have been required to assist with torturous surgical procedures along with having to tend unsightly wounds, and alleviate the suffering of those who were dying painful protracted deaths.

Just a few days after Nurse Alcott arrived at Georgetown there was a huge arrival of wounded Union soldiers. These were the casualties incurred when General Robert E. Lee led the Confederate Army to victory at the imposing Battle of Fredericksburg that had involved almost two hundred thousand troops. As the wounded poured in, Alcott recoiled at the utter magnitude of human suffering the under provisioned staff was expected to contend with. She was so shocked that at first she hid behind a pile of clothing emerging only after she had composed herself. Then she got to work washing away blood and filth. Her experiences and gift for communication would culminate in her literary work and inspire the resoundingly successful semi-autobiographical novel *Little Women*.

Dorothea Lynde Dix had already been widely acknowledged among the medical community of the day as a crusader and reformer. Her actual medical experience and qualifications were questionable but once appointed, her dedication to duty was beyond reproach. The problems facing armies both north and south can't be underestimated. Before the outbreak of the Civil War, the United States had maintained an army of between twenty thousand to twenty-five thousand men. Except in the case of the Mexican War, no authority in the country had ever coped with the problem of dealing with the medical care of forces larger than those of the few regiments quartered in distant parts of the Union. Army nursing was regarded as a wholly male domain.

After the outbreak of hostilities, Dix effectively convinced cynical military officials that women were perfectly capable of doing the job of nursing, and on the basis of this she personally recruited two thousand women and formed the first Army Nursing Corps. Her frequently autocratic, authoritative style earned her the nickname "Dragon Dix,"[69] not a woman to be messed with. Women volunteered their services on both sides of the Mason-Dixon line, but the vast majority were unqualified and totally inexperienced for the tasks they were about to face. Ms. Dix was often at loggerheads with military officials and when it suited, she blatantly ignored military orders. It's an indisputable fact that army nursing care improved substantially under her supervision. She could on occasion be a little tyrannical, but she took good care of the nurses who labored in the most terrible conditions. She even took measures to obtain vital health care supplies from private agencies when the government was not willing to provide them.

At the time of her appointment, Ms. Dix was nearly sixty years old, and not in the best of health. Her constitution had suffered malaria, long punishing hours of work, and pulmonary weakness. Throughout the previous decades she had operated single-handedly planning her own projects, taking her own advice, and pressing on, unhindered by the opinions of others as she strove to improve conditions in jails and mental asylums. Here was a woman reinforced by her own towering idealism, by her thirst for organizational perfection and discipline. Precisely the qualities needed for her recent appointment according to the Union authorities.

So many wounded and sick soldiers flowed into Washington after the Battle of Manassas (1st Bull Run) that Ms. Dix's hospitals couldn't accommodate them all. She quickly requisitioned more buildings and converted them into hospitals to meet with the high demand. When she discovered that the Union troops didn't have sufficient ambulances, she

---

[69] Dorothea Dix: New England Reformer. By Thomas J. Brown.

purchased one with her own money and dispatched it to Manassas. She also took concerted steps to amend the gender pay imbalance because at the time male nurses were paid $20.50 a month and received rations, clothing, and housing. All of Ms. Dix's nurses were unpaid volunteers. When they discovered that their male counterparts were receiving so many financial and material concessions from the government, there was some unrest. Ms. Dix realized that something had to be done, otherwise she was in danger of losing a lot of great nurses. She applied to the governmental authorities and achieved a victory when they agreed to provide the female nurses with food, transportation, and housing. They also agreed to pay the nurses forty cents per day, and thanks to this the nursing staff increased in number. This is where Ms. Dix shone brightly. She was a persuasive and demanding campaigner who had both the intelligence and experience to effectively achieve her goals.

Dorothea Lynde Dix was a pioneer, a reformer who applied herself (heart and soul) to her campaigning work. Her contribution to the Civil War pales by comparison to the reforms she achieved concerning the improvement of care for the mentally ill in America. Thanks to her untiring efforts and the unfathomable depth of her compassion for her cause, the first insane asylums were created. She never stopped campaigning and continued until ill health prevented her. She died in an apartment adjacent to a hospital in New Jersey July 17, 1887.

It's difficult to summarize the age of twenty-seven. In April of 1862, against the express wishes of her family and along with forty other women, Kate Cummings (1828–1909) left for Northern Mississippi. The group of women who were all inexperienced arrived at the perimeter of the battlefield of Shiloh while the battle was still raging. Nothing could have prepared her for the sights and sounds she experienced at seeing the survivors of one Confederate regiment after the battle. She wrote: "When within a few miles of the place, we could realize the condition of an army immediately after a battle. Nothing that I had ever read or heard could have given me the faintest idea of the horrors I witnessed here. I do not think the words are in our vocabulary expressive enough to present to the mind that realities of that sad scene. Certainly none of the glories of the war were presented here. "Gray-haired men- men in the pride of manhood beardless boys, Federals and all mutilated in every imaginable way, lying on the floor, just as they were taken from the battlefield; so close together that it was impossible to walk without stepping on them."

Completely shocked by the experience of tending to battlefield casualties most of the initial group left soon after, but Kate remained in nearby Corinth and Okalona, Mississippi, until June 1862. After that she spent two months in Mobile, Alabama, and thereafter volunteered to work at Newsome Hospital in Chattanooga, Tennessee, where she would remain for a year until the summer of 1863 when the city was evacuated. It was around this time that Confederate government officially recognized the role of women in hospitals. The first time that Kate inadvertently wandered into an amputation room she was deeply distressed by what she saw there: "A stream of blood ran from the table into a tub in which was the arm. It had been taken off at the socket, and the hand, which but a short time before grasped the musket and battled from the right, was hanging over the edge of the tub, a lifeless things [sic]."

After months in the hospital and witnessing similar sights, Kate found herself wishing that she could become more emotionally resilient like some of the other nurses that surrounded her. "I often wish that I could become as callous as many seem to be, for there is no end to these horrors." Becoming emotionally distanced is considered a prerequisite for nurses these days, but for someone who hadn't experienced formal medical training it was tough to mentally detach from the sights, sounds and smells of the immediate environment. Kate Cummings wanted to be more tenacious so that she could prevent becoming visibly upset at the death of soldiers, or being moved by the amount of blood and wounded men in her proximity.

Kate wrote, "Although many were skeptical of letting women give aid to the soldiers, the soldiers themselves were very thankful. If I were to live a hundred years, I should never forget the poor sufferers' gratitude; for every little things [sic] done for them- a little water to drink, or the bathing of their wounds- seemed to afford them the greatest relief." From 1863 until the end of the war, Kate worked in the caravan of mobile field hospitals established throughout Georgia to counteract the effects of General Sherman's devastation. The towns included Kingston, Cherokee Springs, Catoosa Springs, Tunnel Hill, Marietta, and Newnan. Kate's work as a nurse was not particularly extraordinary, but the meticulously detailed journal she kept during the War remains an invaluable testimony to the hardships nurses endured and the almost indescribable suffering of the wounded men in their care.

One of the most distinguished and memorable nurses to emerge from the American Civil War was Clarissa Harlowe Barton (better known simply as Clara Barton). She was an educator, a patent clerk, a nurse, the founder of the American Red Cross, and the youngest of six children. Born Christmas Day, December 1821, in North Oxford, Massachusetts, she was the daughter of farmer Stephen Barton who supported the abolitionist movement and was also a Freemason who firmly believed in the importance of education. Her mother Sarah was an active women's rights campaigner. In her lifetime Clara became known as the "Angel of the Battlefield." She independently organized facilities and secured medicine and supplies for casualties sustained during some of the fiercest battles of that terrible war. Her efforts saved the lives of many men wounded in the Union Army at the battles of Cedar Mountain, Bull Run, Chantilly, Antietam, Fredericksburg, Hilton Head, the Wilderness, and Petersburg.

When the Civil War got underway in 1861 and injured troops arrived after their first major encounter, Clara Barton was there with some other volunteer nurses to receive them and tend to their wounds. As soon as their supply of handkerchiefs was exhausted, she rushed home and tore up her bed sheets to use as bandages. This was her first encounter with superficial war wounds but it wouldn't be her last.

Clara remained fiercely patriotic toward the Union cause and had expressed genuine fears that the Southern aristocracy, by their close combination and superior political training, might succeed in gradually subjugating the whole country. But in her mind, now that the Union had rallied to the flag, that was no longer going to be the case.

Around this time Clara took the initiative to place an advertisement in the newspaper *The Worcester Spy*, requesting stores, supplies, and money for the wounded and needy of the 6th Regiment. She was quite graphic when she stated that she would personally receive and distribute all shipments. The city of Worcester was the first to send assistance, and soon after surrounding towns and cities in Massachusetts followed its example.

The public response was phenomenal. The number of packages that were sent was so great that Clara's room was filled to the rafters and she was obliged to secure space in a nearby warehouse on 7th Street and Pennsylvania Avenue. In the weeks that followed, as more regiments arrived in Washington, she made it her personal duty to supply them with food, medical provisions, and clothing. Due to the glaring lack of any coordinated military organization, the regiments were in desperate need of these supplies. Clara and her associates compensated for this organizational vacuum and worked incredibly hard to establish the shipping and distribution of supplies. She appears to have discovered a serious purpose to her life, a meaning that transcended the desultory offices and schoolrooms that she had previously been associated with.

Throughout the following weeks and months, she began meeting the wounded soldiers disembarking at the dockside after returning on the transports from the swamps of the Chickahominy in the Peninsular Campaign. She personally saw congealed blood and swamp clay thickly encrusted on terrible wounds and men delirious with pain. Clara did what she could to ease their suffering, applying warm water, lotions, and clean dressings. She labored hard tending these men amid the flies and filth, surrounded by festering sores and putrid odors, under the sweltering Maryland sun. When one batch was transported off to hospital, another arrived on a seemingly endless production line of human misery. Most women of the day would have probably fainted at these abhorrent sights and smells. Clara had discovered her *raison d'etre*, her chosen métier and she applied great vehemence and professionalism to her task.

Reflecting on her service during the Civil war in later years she wrote: "I was strong and thought I might go to the rescue of the men who fell. The first regiment of troops, the old 6th Mass. that fought its way through Baltimore, brought my playmates and neighbors, the partakers of my childhood, the brigades of New Jersey brought scores of my brave boys, the same solid phalanx; and the strongest legions from old Herkimer brought the associates of my seminary days. They formed and crowded around me. What could I do but go with them, or work for them and my country? The patriot blood of my father was warm in my veins. But I struggled long and hard with my sense of propriety, with the appalling fact that I was only a woman whispering in one ear, and thundering in the other the groans of suffering men dying like dogs, unfed and unsheltered, for the life of every institution which had protected and educated me! I said that I struggled with my sense of propriety and I say it with humiliation and shame. I am ashamed that I thought of such a thing."[70]

Places such as Fair Oaks and Cedar Mountain that have since become ingrained in Civil War history.

Later on she wrote: "When our armies fought on Cedar Mountain, I broke the shackles and went to the field. Five days and nights with three hours sleep, a narrow escape from capture and some days of getting the wounded into hospitals at Washington brought Saturday, August 30. And if you chance to feel, that the positions I occupied were rough and unseemly for a woman I can only reply that they were rough and unseemly for men. But under all, lay the life of the nation. I had inherited the rich blessing of health and strength of constitution such as are seldom given to woman, and I felt that some return was due from me and that I ought to be there."[71]

Eighteen-sixty-two was a seminal year in the life of Clara Barton, undeterred by the warnings and spurred by her singularity of purpose; by late August, she began providing direct battlefield assistance. The reluctant generals eventually provided her with passes on the premise that she had given them her personal assurance that she would neither run nor complain if she was in the line of fire. This forty-one-year-old spinster must have been aware that she was embarking on a course that

---

[70] A Quiet Will: The Life of Clara Barton (Abridged, Annotated). By William E. Barton.

[71] The Life of Clara Barton, Founder of the American Red Cross, Volume 1. By W.E. Barton.

would entail great risk to both herself and her associates, moreover the horrors of mid–19th century warfare made that a difficult vow to sustain.

Civil War medical procedures such as amputations in proximity to the battlefield were common, and incurred a 27 percent mortality rate among Union troops. Although surgeons generally used ether or chloroform as an anesthetic, and despite many surgical advances being made during the war, antiseptic surgery was still in its infancy, and consequently many soldiers perished due to infection. Chloroform was first used as an anesthetic in 1847. Because it allowed surgeons to perform painful operations more slowly, they could better prepare amputation stumps for prostheses. By the time the American Civil War broke out in 1861, both ether and chloroform had been in use for several years as methods of surgical anesthesia. Though both anesthetic agents were developed around the 1840s, chloroform soon emerged as the more ubiquitously applied anesthetic because it worked faster than ether and was non-flammable. During the Civil War, ether (and particularly chloroform) became indispensable tools for military doctors who performed tens of thousands of amputations and other types of procedures for wounded Union and Confederate soldiers.

In 1862 Clara Barton witnessed the Battle of Antietam and was present at one of the bloodiest and most devastating battles of the whole American Civil War. She recalled an incident that would have unnerved the most steadfast: "A man lying upon the ground asked for a drink, I stopped to give it, and having raised him with my right hand, was holding him. Just at this moment a bullet sped its free and easy way between us, tearing a hole in my sleeve and found its way into his body. He fell back dead. There was no more to be done for him and I left him to his rest. I have never mended that hole in my sleeve."[72]

By the end of the battle, Clara had contracted a fever of such severity she was unable to walk unaided; however, this didn't prevent her from complaining bitterly to Quartermaster General Rucker that she could have done more if her supplies hadn't been exhausted. Rucker gave

---

[72] The Life of Clara Barton, Founder of the American Red Cross, Volume 1. By W.E. Barton.

his personal assurance that this would never be the case again. Union General Benjamin Butler was so impressed by Clara's tenacity and courage that he officially appointed her as the "lady in charge" of the hospitals.

Both Union and Confederate armies experienced indescribable suffering at the Battle of Antietam. After three days of violent combat, it produced the single bloodiest day in American history culminating in the deaths of 12,410 Union and 10,700 Confederate soldiers. Although militarily it ended without a decisive victory for either side, the fact that Lee had retreated back over the river was enough for the North to proclaim it as a success. More importantly it was a propaganda victory for the North because the war now obtained a dual purpose. Apart from preserving the Union, five days after the Battle of Antietam, President Lincoln used it as a catalyst to issue his "Emancipation Proclamation,"[73] stating that all slaves held in rebelling states were to be freed on January 1, 1863.

During the final year of the war, Clara was informed of the vast number of MIAs that had accumulated throughout the previous four years. She received letters from various parts of the country, stating that a significant number of soldiers had disappeared without a trace. Concerned relatives of the missing had no idea what had become of their loved ones, whether they had fallen in battle, were suffering in Confederate POW camps, or had perished in some other way that they could only speculate. On the strength of this, in the spring of 1865, Clara took it upon herself to personally assist in discovering the fates of some these men. She began by distributing printed lists of MIAs to be displayed in conspicuous places, requesting information from anyone who may be able to help. Using her skill as an administrator, she initiated and organized a government-supported department that dealt with up to one hundred letters a day. On the basis of this she made a nationwide appeal for information that became eminently popular with the public and produced significant results. Clara and her assistants received and answered more than sixty-three thousand letters and identified over twenty-two thousand missing men.

---

[73] The Emancipation Proclamation: Ending Slavery in America. By Adam Woog.

One Union soldier named Dorence Atwater who had been a POW at the notorious Confederate prison at Andersonville secretly made an official list of the dead and their burial. During his incarceration he had hidden the list of more than thirteen thousand names in his coat lining. Forty-five thousand Union soldiers suffered unimaginable horrors while being held. During the worst months, one hundred men died each day from malnutrition, exposure to the elements, and communicable disease. After the war Andersonville commandant Captain Henry Wirz was arrested and found guilty by a military tribunal. He was hanged in Washington, D.C., November 10, 1865, and was the only person executed for war crimes during the Civil War.

In the fall of 1869 Clara decided to observe her doctor's advice and travel to Europe for three years rest. While visiting Geneva she heard about a book written by a Mr. Henry Dunant, entitled *Un Souvenir de Solferino (A Memory of Solferino),*[74] which inspired the establishment of the "Geneva Convention" and the Red Cross organization. Dunant had witnessed the tragic aftermath of the Battle of Solferino firsthand when he toured the area the day after it occurred. Solferino was a particularly bloody encounter where forty thousand men were killed or wounded in just fifteen intense, ferocious hours of fighting. In 1862 he published his observations. Readers were shocked by Dunant's vivid and graphic descriptions of the violence and brutality of armed conflict. They were equally moved by his account of the plight of the wounded and of the noble but pitifully inadequate efforts that he and his little band of helpers had made to alleviate the suffering. His proposals for ameliorating the condition of the wounded in future wars so impressed the European public and many well-placed supporters that he had no problem raising volunteers and gaining support for his organization.

On July 19, 1870, four days after France had declared war on Prussia (hailing the outbreak of the Franco-Prussian War), officials from the International Red Cross of Europe approached Clara Barton, who at that time was still in Switzerland recuperating. This was one of the many

---

[74] A Memory of Solferino. By Henri Dunant.

factors that gave Clara the impetus to establish the Red Cross in America. She wrote, "As I journeyed on and saw the work of these Red Cross societies in the field, accomplishing in four months under their systematic organization what we failed to accomplish in four years without it no mistakes, no needless suffering, no starving, no lack of care, no waste, no confusion, but order, plenty, cleanliness and comfort wherever that little flag made its way a whole continent marshaled under the banner of the Red Cross, as I saw all this, and joined and worked in it, you will not wonder that I said to myself 'if I live to return to my country I will try to make my people understand the Red Cross and that treaty.' But I did more than resolve, I promised other nations I would do it, and other reasons pressed me to remember my promise."[75]

In 1877, Clara lobbied President Rutherford B. Hayes in an attempt to procure his endorsement of the Geneva Convention. Hayes expressed interest at first, but had serious reservations regarding the treaty's connotations that he regarded as a "possible entangling alliance" with European nations. This prompted him to ultimately reject her petition. Impervious to this rejection, Clara established the American Red Cross and held the first meeting in her Washington apartment on May 21, 1881. She paved the way, displayed incredible courage and fortitude, and it's for these and many other qualities that this battlefield angel deserves to be remembered. She died at her home in Glen Echo, Maryland, in 1912 at the grand old age of ninety-one.

Captain Sally Louisa Tompkins is said to be the only woman ever to receive a military commission from the Confederate Army during the American Civil War. Many regard her as America's first female army officer, but this claim has never been definitively ascertained. She was in many respects the Southern counterpart to the North's Clara Barton. Sally came into the world November 9, 1833, at Poplar Grove in Mathews County, Virginia. By 1854 the same year her mother had passed away, Sally moved to Richmond, Virginia. Shortly after the first battle of Manassas (Bull Run) she established the Robertson Hospital

---

[75] Clara Barton: In the Service of Humanity. By David Henry Burton.

at the home of Judge John Robertson on Main Street in Richmond. It only had twenty-two beds at its disposal but this number was frequently exceeded. Standing at a diminutive five feet tall, she became known to the confederates as the "Little Lady with the Milk-White Hands." In Sally's case size didn't matter one iota because she attended her duties with a level of vivacity and determination that astounded and endeared many of her patients.

Shortly after Sally opened her hospital, Confederate Surgeon General Samuel P. Moore determined that extensive military hospitals with commissioned officers should replace the many private hospitals, which in his opinion, with all the best will in the world couldn't provide their patients with sufficient care. When it came to the attention of Jefferson Davis that Robertson Hospital had the highest number of previously wounded returning to duty, he commissioned Sally as a captain on September 9, 1861, and decided to keep her hospital open. She flatly refused any kind of payment for her service and when she was commissioned, she wrote, "I accepted the above commission as Captain in the CSA when it was offered. But, I would not allow my name to be placed upon the pay roll of the army." Robertson Hospital remained operative until June 1865, when the last patients were discharged.

Thanks to a substantial inheritance left to her by her late father before the war, she personally funded the hospital in the beginning, but according to various editions of the "Richmond Dispatch," she also readily accepted donations from patriotic and philanthropic sources that actively supported the southern cause.

It was alleged that the hospital had the lowest death rate of any Civil War hospital North or South of the Mason Dixon line, and some even say that due to this the Confederate Army sent her the most difficult cases. Throughout the whole Civil War only 73 patients out of more than 1,330 admitted died while in her care, but statistics vary. The Confederate government sent a number of qualified doctors to assist her. Among these was Dr. Alexander Yelverton Peyron Garnett who was appointed as her head surgeon and provided much needed food and supplies. Among other things, Garnett personally attended to General Robert E. Lee and his family during the war along with several members of the Confederate Congress and cabinet and other Confederate generals.

It's no secret that Garnett didn't like Captain Sally, and they didn't get along well at all. Due to his misogynistic attitude, he found it problematic accepting her rank and authority, but this didn't stop her from being assertive when it came to the care of her adoring patients. Ten years after the war ended, she remained in Richmond and later moved to the home of John Lightfoot and Harriet Field Lightfoot in Port Royal, Virginia. Sally bought the property in November 1896 and owned it until 1905. After eventually exhausting her inheritance, she spent the remaining years of her life at the "Home for Needy Confederate Women in Richmond." Captain Sally Louisa Tompkins died July 25, 1916, at the age of eighty-three and was buried with full military honors at Kingston Episcopal Parish Church cemetery in Mathews County, Virginia.

It is fitting and appropriate that this chapter should end with the contribution made by former African American slave Susie King Taylor. She was born into slavery on August 6, 1848, at the Great Plantation in Liberty County in coastal Georgia. Her mother was a domestic servant.

At a time when it was strictly forbidden for slaves to learn to read and write, at the tender age of seven her owner allowed her to live with her grandmother Dolly in Savannah, Georgia. It has even been suggested that her owner may have purposefully released her from bondage. In Savannah Susie surreptitiously attended to two schools secretly run by African American women who taught her to read and write. At that time clandestine schooling was the only way an African American child could get an education in the Antebellum South. At the age of thirteen, Susie King Taylor escaped from slavery and by the time the Civil War broke out in 1861 she was an educated, erudite young woman whose abilities had surpassed the level of knowledge provided by her first teachers in Georgia. A Union army commander asked her to start a school for children who, like her, had escaped slavery with their families. She ran a small school at each army camp she went to. While serving in the army she met the notable Ms. Clara Barton. When the war reached its conclusion, Susie was hoping to continue teaching but despite her efforts, she encountered many difficulties.

Eventually Susie got a job as a domestic servant, but in her memoirs she wrote that her "interest in the boys in blue had not abated." Taylor also dedicated much of her postwar life to helping veterans and their families. She joined the Women's Relief Corps, Auxiliary to the Grand Army of the Republic, and organized Corps 67. She died in October 1912.

Her personal memoirs are the only known published recollections of an African American nurse during the Civil War. She taught free blacks and former slaves. She served the 33rd Regiment of the United States Colored Troops for more than three years, alongside her husband, Edward King, a sergeant in the regiment. Like many African American nurses, Taylor was never paid for her work as a nurse during the Civil War.

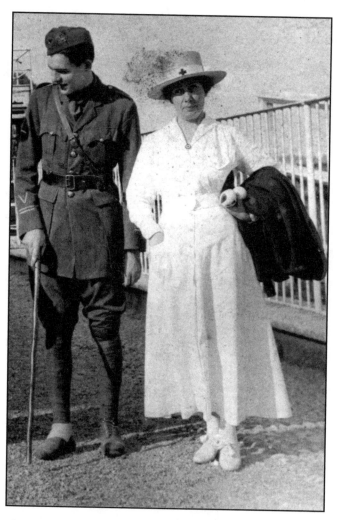

Agnes von Kurowsky—the Philadelphia-native Red Cross nurse treated future writer Ernest Hemingway in Italy during World War I and was the inspiration for Catherine Barkley in Hemingway's book *A Farewell to Arms.*

Courtesy of National Archives

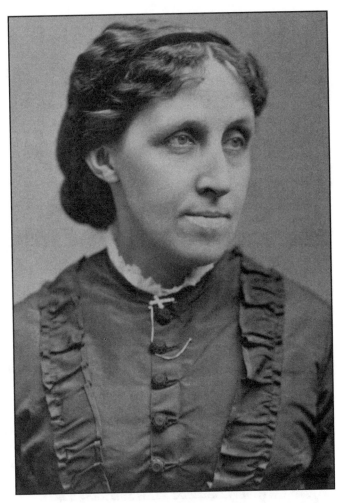

Louisa May Alcott—abolitionist, feminist, and Civil
War nurse who served in a hospital in Georgetown
Washington, D.C. in 1862–1863 and went on
to write the acclaimed novel *Little Women*.

Courtesy of Library of Congress

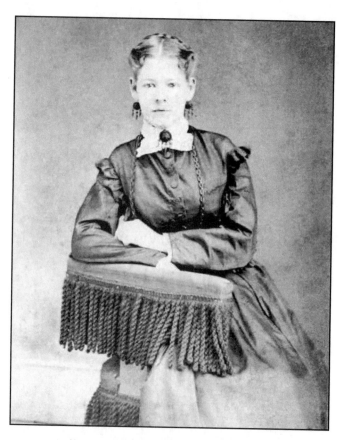

Tillie Pierce—she was well known for her firsthand account of the Battle of Gettysburg, *At Gettysburg, or, What a Girl Saw and Heard of the Battle: A True Narrative* and she later on assisted as a nurse at Gettysburg's Camp Letterman General Hospital in August, 1863.

Courtesy of Library of Congress

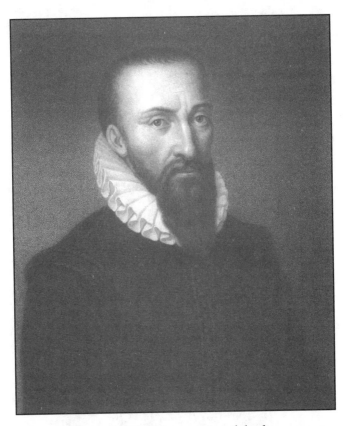

Ambroise Pare—a 16th Century French barber surgeon
who many regard as the father of modern surgery,
pathology, and battlefield medicine as well. He sought
to help soothe the patient along with treating their
wound or affliction, which was unheard of at the time.

Courtesy of CORBIS

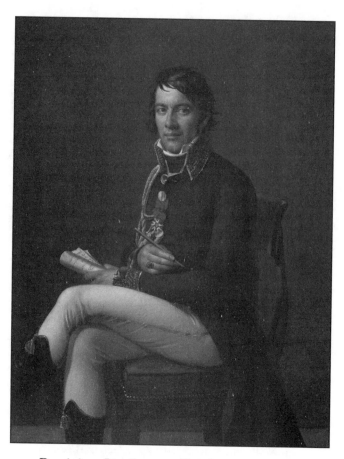

Dominique Jean Larrey—Napolean Bonaparte's
favorite doctor, and the father of modern military
surgery, Larrey established revolutionary
amputation methods, encouraged the role of nurses
on the battlefield, and mobile triage units.

Courtesy of Augustins Museum

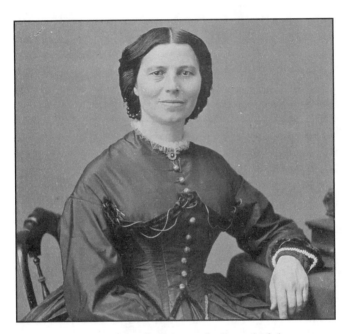

Clara Barton—known as the "angel of the battlefield" during the American Civil War, Barton did not have formal medical training but her efforts saved countless lives. She helped with the formation of the American Red Cross.

Courtesy of Library of Congress

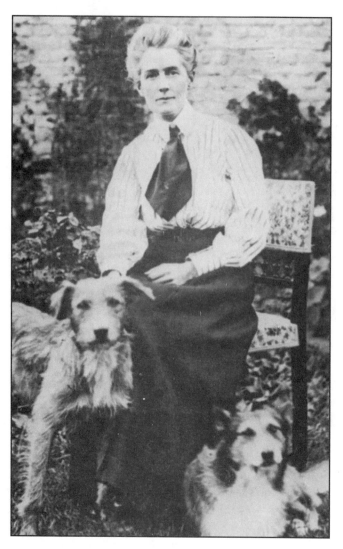

Edith Cavell—British World War I nurse, who treated both sides during the conflict but also assisted with the escape of Allied soldiers from Belgium, which resulted in her arrest by German authorities and execution.

Courtesy of CORBIS

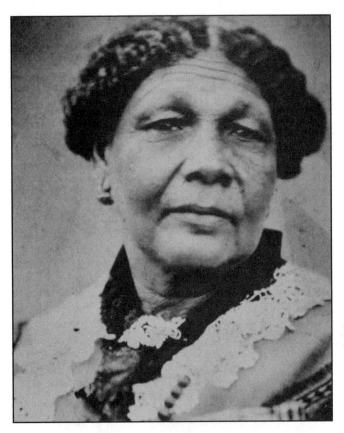

Mary Seacole—British-Jamaican nurse during the Crimean War who set up the "British Hotel" behind the lines and using her knowledge of medicine during her travels, set up a place to help wounded officers. She also went out onto the battlefield to treat wounded soldiers too.

Courtesy of National Geographic

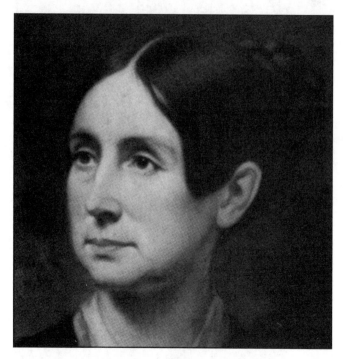

Dorothea Dix—American Civil War nurse who
was appointed the Superintendent of Army
Nurses for the Union Army, which appointed
thousands of nurses and treated both Union and
Confederation casualties during the war.

Courtesy of Library of Congress

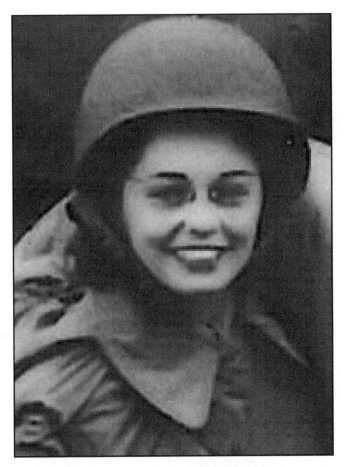

Dorothy Barre—American World War II nurse
who served with the 16th General Hospital in
Liege, Belgium throughout her time in World War
II. She treated many survivors of the Battle of the
Bulge and faced repeated V1 Buzz Bomb attacks
along with enemy aircraft attacks as well.

Courtesy of Dorothy Barre

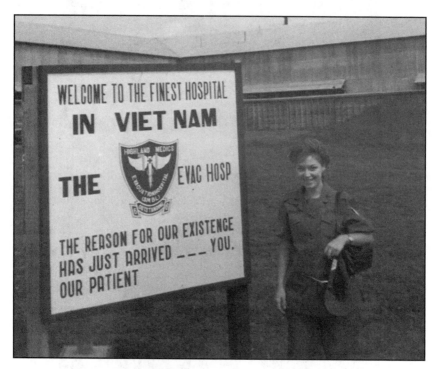

Mary "Edie" Meeks—American Vietnam War nurse
who served in the U.S. Army, is pictured outside of the
71st Evacuation Hospital in Pleiku, Vietnam.

Courtesy of Mary "Edie" Meeks

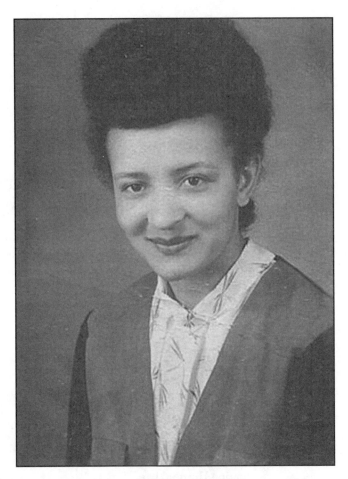

Augusta Chiwy—a Belgian-Congolese nurse who
volunteered to treat American soldiers in Bastogne,
Belgium during the Battle of the Bulge and was later
knighted by the Belgian government for her service.

Courtesy of Augusta Chiwy

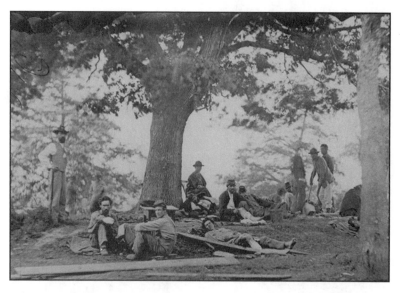

Wounded soldiers during the American Civil War faced frightening
conditions in field hospitals, but for many it was the waiting to be
taken off the battlefield that was just as painful as their treatment.

Courtesy of National Archives

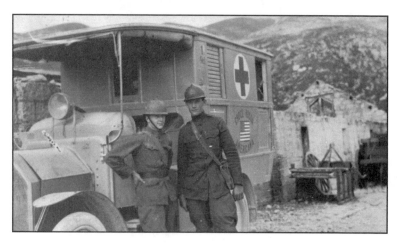

The United States did not enter World War I until 1917 but the
American Volunteer Ambulance Service went over to France in
1914 to set up hospitals and medical services. The Ambulance
Service continued to be an independent unit until the U.S. Army
took over when the United States joined the Allied cause.

Courtesy of National Archives

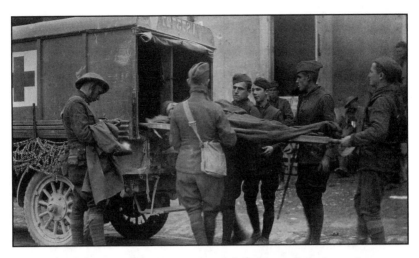

World War I introduced unique and difficult wounds due to heavy artillery, gas attacks, and deadlier machine guns. Medical technology also evolved with better medicine, medical knowledge, and transportation.

Courtesy of National Archives

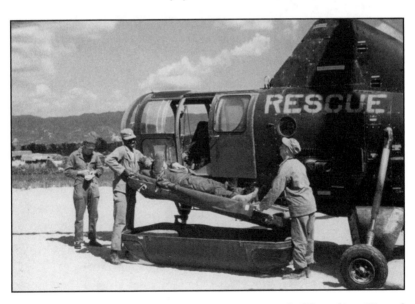

MEDEVAC missions became paramount to survival of front line GIs and Marines during the Korean Conflict, the helicopters were nicknamed the "Angels of Mercy" by the wounded who were evacuated.

Courtesy of National Archives

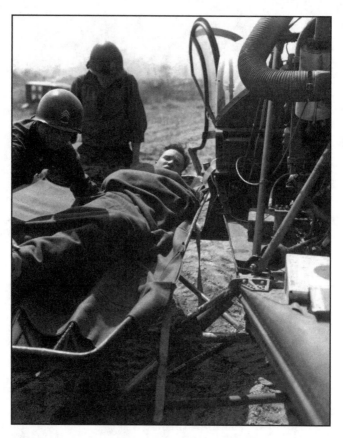

Evacuation of soldiers from the frontlines in helicopters became a major part of the Korean Conflict. Here, a wounded GI is put on a stretcher to be flown out to a MASH unit for treatment. Medical treatment during the Vietnam War became even more streamlined with improved MEDEVAC and field hospital operations which were brought back to U.S. hospitals too.

Courtesy of National Archives

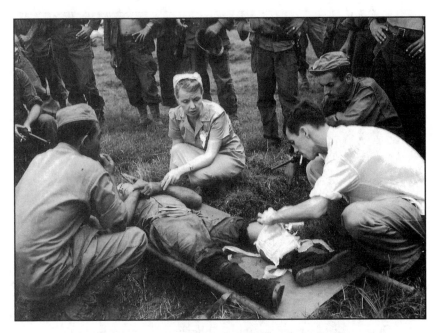

Nurses became a major part of medical care in the Vietnam
War and helped with the mass casualties that were coming
into the field hospitals and main hospitals.

Courtesy of National Archives

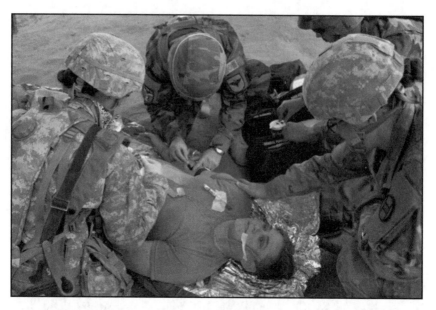

The Wars in Iraq and Afghanistan began a new era of survivability
for American service members. Bullet and trauma wounds that
would have killed a World War II GI in 1942 were now able
to be treated and allow the service member to survive through
technology and even better MEDEVAC operations.

Courtesy of the U.S. Army

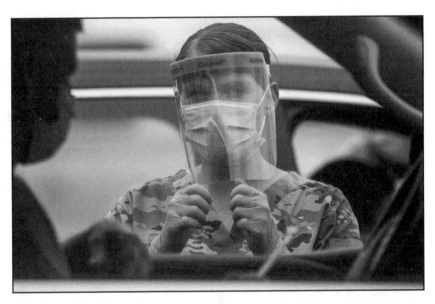

During the COVID-19 pandemic, National Guard members throughout the U.S. assisted with the distribution of PPE (Personal Protection Equipment) and with testing. Pfc. Kelly Buterbaugh, a combat medic with the Delaware National Guard, is shown administering a test to a member of the public.

Courtesy of U.S. National Guard

PART 2

INNOVATIONS

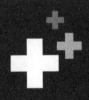

CHAPTER TWELVE

Cavell and the Americans

The American Minister to Belgium during the Great War was Brand Whitlock. Celebrated as a great American author, accomplished attorney, and four-term mayor of Toledo, Ohio, he earned the nickname "*Le Ministre Protecteur*" (minister protector) because of his role as an advocate for Belgian citizens and condemned prisoners in German occupied Belgium. It was because of this that his name would become inextricably linked to the fate of British nurse Edith Cavell. But did he really do everything he could to save her life? The answer to that is that he did everything within his remit. The intransigent German authorities had taken the decision to execute Edith Cavell for her indiscretions, and no diplomatic power on earth would be able to prevent that.

History records Edith Cavell as a British nurse and humanitarian. So much has been written about her throughout the decades that it has become difficult to extract the person from the legend. It's a fact that the intrinsic propaganda value of her death to British authorities during World War One was incalculable. But it's controversial to suggest that she was worth more to them dead than alive, although this is entirely possible.

Since 1915, disseminated by books, articles and films, the legend of this whiter than white, courageous nurse Cavell has continued to grow. There were few war heroes who received as many posthumous tributes as Nurse Cavell, and there were few incidents during World War One that provoked as much indignation and outrage as the execution of this seemingly innocuous nurse. She has been described as a martyr, a saint, a legendary figure who was cruelly executed by Germans. It's all very black and white, maybe too clean cut. She was grace and kindness incarnate and the Germans were evil and depraved. But was it all that straightforward?

In the wee small hours October 12, 1915, long before the first hesitant rays of dawn permeated the overcast sky, two cars trundled over uneven cobbled streets toward the Brussels suburb of Schaerbeek. One of them was transporting a British nurse to her place of execution. Just a few months prior on August 4, 1915, a year after Britain had declared war on Germany, Nurse Edith Cavell was arrested in Brussels, accused and found guilty by a German military tribunal of having played an active role in helping Allied soldiers to escape occupied Belgium. Being a painfully honest person, she never denied the charges and was held in solitary confinement in St. Gilles Prison in Brussels until she attended a trial that lasted just two days in 1915: Thursday, October seventh, and Friday, October eighth. After a further weekend in solitary confinement, at 4:30 p.m. on Monday, October eleventh, Edith Cavell was sentenced to death by firing squad.

The Germans had accumulated sufficient evidence implicating Edith Cavell as being involved, but not the leader of an underground organization. Moreover, she had freely admitted her guilt. General von Bissing had no interest in granting clemency despite the fact that executing a Red Cross nurse had the potential to stir up violent emotions and a cycle of blame that would inevitably denounce Germany.

Now, as then, there was a darker purpose. Apart from other things, Edith's death deflected attention away from the CRB (Commission for Relief of Belgium) and its role in providing food for the German army, a role which Belgian historians seem determined to suppress. The

CRB was the parent organization of the Belgian American Educational Foundation, established October 1914 by American Herbert Hoover. A group of prominent Belgians and Americans residing in Belgium had approached the American Ambassador to Great Britain to organize measures of relief in the face of terrible food shortages in Belgium.

Hugh Simons made much of his remonstrations with the German administration on the eve of Edith Cavell's execution, but Gibson was first and foremost a Hoover man, and was merely following protocol, going through the motions. There were some notable Belgians who openly resented Hoover's interference in Belgian affairs on a personal level, but it is debatable whether any one individual could have taken effective steps at the last minute to save Edith Cavell. The most damning accusation is that Edith Cavell's death probably suited the needs of the CRB. Hugh Gibson wrote a report addressed to the Secretary of U.S. Legation to Belgium American Legation, Brussels. October 12, 1915:

> *"Sir,*
>
> *Upon learning early yesterday morning through unofficial sources that the trial of Miss Edith Cavell had been finished on Saturday afternoon, and that the prosecuting attorney ("Kriegsgerichtsrat") had asked for a sentence of death against her, telephonic inquiry was immediately made at the Politische Abteilung as to the facts.*
>
> *"It was stated that no sentence had as yet been pronounced and that there would probably be delay of a day or two before a decision was reached. Mr. Conrad gave positive assurances that the Legation would be fully informed as to developments in this case.*
>
> *"Despite these assurances, we made repeated inquiries in the course of the day, the last one being at 6.20 p.m. Belgian time. Mr. Conrad then stated that sentence had not yet been pronounced, and specifically renewed his previous*

assurances that he would not fail to inform us as soon as there was any news.

"At 8.30 it was learned from an outside source that sentence had been passed in the course of the afternoon (before the last conversation with Mr. Conrad), and that the execution would take place during the night.

"In conformity with your instructions, I went (accompanied by Mr. de Leval) to look for the Spanish Minister and found him dining at the home of Baron Lambert. I explained the circumstances to his Excellency and asked that (as you were ill and unable to go yourself) he go with us to see Baron von der Lancken and support as strongly as possible the plea, which I was to make in your name, that execution of the death penalty should be deferred until the Governor could consider your appeal for clemency.

"We took with us a note addressed to Baron von der Lancken, and a plea for clemency ("requete en grace") addressed to the Governor-General. The Spanish Minister willingly agreed to accompany us, and we went together to the Politische Abteilung.

"Baron von der Lancken and all the members of his staff were absent for the evening. We sent a messenger to ask that he return at once to see us in regard to a matter of utmost urgency.

"A little after 10 o'clock he arrived, followed shortly after by Count Harrach and Herr von Falkenhausen, members of his staff. The circumstances of the case were explained to him and your note presented, and he read it aloud in our presence.

"He expressed disbelief in the report that sentence had actually been passed, and manifested some surprise that we should give credence to any report not emanating from official sources. He was quite insistent on knowing the exact source of our information, but this I did not feel at liberty to communicate to him.

"Baron von der Lancken stated that it was quite improbable that sentence had been pronounced, that even if so, it would not be executed within so short a time, and that in any event it would be quite impossible to take any action before morning. It was, of course, pointed out to him that if the facts were as we believed them to be, action would be useless unless taken at once. We urged him to ascertain the facts immediately, and this, after some hesitancy, he agreed to do.

"He telephoned to the presiding judge of the court-martial and returned in a short time to say that the facts were as we had represented them, and that it was intended to carry out the sentence before morning.

"We then presented, as earnestly as possible, your plea for delay. So far as I am able to judge, we neglected to present no phase of the matter which might have had any effect, emphasizing the horror of executing a woman, no matter what her offence, pointing out that the death sentence had heretofore been imposed only for actual cases of espionage, and that Miss Cavell was not even accused by the German authorities of anything so serious.

"I further called attention to the failure to comply with Mr. Conrad's promise to inform the Legation of the sentence. I urged that inasmuch as the offences charged against Miss Cavell were long since accomplished, and that as she had *been for some weeks in prison, a delay in carrying out the sentence could entail no danger to the German cause.*

"I even went so far as to point out the fearful effect of a summary execution of this sort upon public opinion, both here and abroad, and, although I had no authority for doing so, called attention to the possibility that it might bring about reprisals.

"The Spanish Minister forcibly supported all our representations and made an earnest plea for clemency.

"Baron von der Lancken stated that the Military Governor was the supreme authority ("Gerichtsherr") in matters of this sort; that appeal from his decision could be carried only to the Emperor, the Governor-General having no authority to intervene in such cases.

"He added that under the provisions of German martial law the Military Governor had discretionary power to accept or to refuse acceptance of an appeal for clemency. After some discussion he agreed to call the Military Governor on to the telephone and learn whether he had already ratified the sentence, and whether there was any chance for clemency.

"He returned in about half an hour, and stated that he had been to confer personally with the Military Governor, who said that he had acted in the case of Miss Cavell only after mature deliberation; that the circumstances in her case were of such a character that he considered the infliction of the death penalty imperative; and that in view of the circumstances of this case he must decline to accept your plea for clemency, or any representation in regard to the matter."[76]

---

[76] The Lansing Papers, 1914-1920. By United States Department of State.

Gaston de Leval was wrongly described by the *New York Times* as the "legal advisor to Edith Cavell." It inferred that Edith had been given legal counsel, but the fact is that she was never properly represented by those charged with her safety, and didn't have any contact with Leval at any given time. Leval was a sycophant, a company man who played a major part in concocting the impression that Brand Whitlock and his American associates had attempted by every avenue to save Cavell from the firing squad. Leval was invited to address a meeting of the Secret Elite's inner sanctum in New York, the Pilgrims of America, on January 26, 1916, at which Lord Bryce, author of the Bryce Report on German Atrocities in Belgium, was present.

The German authorities were infuriated by the negative propaganda that resulted from Cavell's execution. Posters were pasted on the streets of Brussels denying that Whitlock had been kept ignorant regarding the pronunciation of Cavell's death sentence, or that the German Authorities, by proceeding rapidly, had prevented him from intervening in favor of the accused. The official version of events published and approved by the British Foreign Office was condemned as being utterly fallacious. Brand Whitlock stuck to his story, but received permission from Washington to issue Gaston de Leval with an American passport to urgently get him out of Belgium. After all, they could hardly have allowed him to be interrogated by the secret police.

The fallout did not stop with de Leval's surreptitious expulsion. The Germans would never forgive Gibson for his skeptical account of Edith Cavell's trial. He effectively became persona non grata to them. Though he lingered at the Brussels's legation, antagonism to him steadily grew until February 7, 1916, when Von der Lanken arrived at Brand Whitlock's door and demanded that Gibson leave "today or at the latest, tomorrow."[77] The reason noted by Whitlock was quite specific. It was because of Gibson's firm stand in the Edith Cavell affair and ensuing statements, which had now resulted in a crisis. It felt desirable to give him leave of

---

[77] Prolonging the Agony: How The Anglo-American Establishment Deliberately Extended WWI by Three-and-a-Half Years. By Jim Macgregor and Gerry Docherty (TrineDay, 2018).

absence. Whitlock made no serious protest about the loss of his secretary. In this intricate web of complicity, Hugh Gibson, a young ambitious man whose demeanor appealed greatly to Hoover had proved his loyalty to the CRB, found himself promoted to the American Embassy in London. Hoover personally arranged the prestigious appointment.

The British government has always vigorously refuted German claims that Cavell was a spy, but during her actual trial they remained ominously inert for the duration. According to a former director general of MI5, apart from assisting allied soldiers escape occupied Belgium, the British nurse really did help to smuggle out intelligence. Recent discoveries in Belgian archives revealed strong evidence that clearly incriminates Cavell and exposes the dichotomy of her clandestine network. One young Belgian mining engineer (who smuggled British soldiers to Cavell's organization in 1914) was sentenced to fifteen years hard labor for his activities. In his letters he graphically described how he provided the organization with intelligence on German military operations, information about German trench systems, ammunition dumps, and the whereabouts of enemy aircraft.

Edith Cavell was allegedly aware of this information and passed it on through secret channels to the British intelligence services. She wasn't as innocent as the British press claimed back in the day. On the other hand, it's difficult to ascertain precisely how proactive she was within the organization. She knew how to relay secret messages, and it's been conclusively proven that key members of her network were in contact with the Secret Service Bureau, the precursor to MI6, and other Allied intelligence agencies. General Moritz Von Bissing, the German military governor of Belgium who signed the warrant for Cavell's execution, maintained that far from being the innocent victim of circumstances, she gave her full compliance to the espionage operation.

Throughout World War I German occupation authorities in Belgium arrested hundreds of women for participating in espionage. These activities were described as treason and, depending on the severity of the charge, they were punishable by forced labor or execution. Of the ten women who were arrested in Belgium and Northern France between 1914 and 1918, six were Belgian, three were French, and one was British.

Edith Louisa Cavell was born into a devoutly religious family in Swardeston, Norfolk December 4, 1865. Her parents were Reverend Frederick Cavell, an Anglican vicar, and Louisa Sophia Cavell. Previous to Frederick Cavell's appointment in Swardeston, he was curate of St. Mark's, Tollington Park, and before that held a similar position at St. Mary's in the London suburb of Islington. Faith played a vitally important role in Edith's life, and despite the family's meager income, they were all active in local charities. She was the eldest of four children who first attended Norwich High School, and then went on to continue her education at three different boarding schools.

In 1886, she became a governess for a vicar's family in Essex. Two years later, she travelled to Europe visiting Austria, France, and Germany. It was during this European excursion that she began to develop her humanitarian instincts. She donated money to a hospital in Bavaria for the purchase of medical equipment and for her generosity she became known as the "English Angel." It was around this time that she began to develop an active interest in the nursing profession. At Laurel Court, the last boarding school she had attended in England, she had learned to speak French fluently. On the strength of this in 1890, her former head teacher Margaret Gibson recommended her for the post of governess to the François family in Brussels. This was the start of Edith Cavell's enduring but often unreciprocated love affair with Belgium and the Belgian people, but she had some reservations. The matriarch of the family occasionally asked Ms. Cavell to tell visitors that she wasn't home, but Cavell couldn't comply with this request on the basis that she was incapable of telling a lie, something that didn't trouble some duplicitous Belgians.

She graduated as a qualified nurse in September the following year and accepted a position at the London Hospital where she was eventually promoted to staff nurse. She remained there until December 1899. In 1907, Dr. Antoine Depage, a Belgian physician and hospital director, persuaded Cavell to accept a position as Matron at a recently opened nursing school: the *L'École Belge d'Infirmières Diplômées* (The Berkendael

Medical Institute) in a suburb of Brussels. At a time when most Belgian hospitals were staffed by nuns and firmly attached to various religious orders, nurses who were not part of the religious establishment were unjustly vilified as being women of dubious reputation. Dr. Depage wanted to veer the institute away from traditional religious-based care and make it a more secular, science-oriented organization. During her brief career in Belgium, she succeeded in modernizing the standard of Belgian nursing and gained wide recognition for her work. She helped train many nurses who went on to staff other hospitals, nursing homes, and schools around the country, including the clinic at the foreboding St. Gilles Prison, a place that she would get to know better later on. Edith Cavell felt that she had found her place in world and was delighted at the opportunity to teach her chosen profession to young Belgian student nurses.

She wrote: "One of our first duties was to recruit the nurses. The old idea that it is a disgrace for women to work is still held in Belgium, and women of good birth and education still think they lose caste by earning their own living. The contrast the probationers present to the nurses in their heavy stiff robes, and the lay nurses in their grimy apparel, is the contrast of the unhygienic past with the enlightened present. These Belgian probationers have goodwill, courage, and perseverance, and in three years' time they will look back on the first days of trial with wonder. The spread of light and knowledge is bound to follow in years to come. The nurses will not only teach, as none others have the opportunity of doing, the laws of health and the prevention and healing of disease, they will show their countrywomen that education and position do not constitute a bar to an independent life, they are rather a good and solid foundation on which to build a career which demands the best and highest qualities that womanhood can offer."[78] In 1909 she visited England as a delegate to the International Council of Nurses held in London. Her description of the work she was attempting to conduct in Brussels made a deep and lasting impression on the other delegates.

---

[78] Nursing Mirror and Midwives, Volume 160, Issues 14-26 (IPC Specialist and Professional Press, 1985).

Her father died in 1910. When war broke out in 1914, Cavell was in England visiting her mother and other members of her family, and despite their vehement protests, they failed to persuade her to remain in England. Consequently, she decided to return to Belgium to continue her work. She defended this decision when writing to a friend, "My duty is with my nurses."[79]

August fourth was a seminal date in Belgian history. The German army ignored Belgium's neutrality and invaded the country just days after Cavell's return to Brussels. It was the culmination of the domino effect that had started with the assassination of Archduke Ferdinand in Sarajevo. Britain had guaranteed Belgium's neutrality and consequently felt obliged to declare war on Germany for this infraction. Edith Cavell joined the Red Cross, and the Berkendael Institute where she worked was converted into a Red Cross hospital for wounded soldiers of all incumbent nations. Even though Cavell was a citizen of an enemy nation, German military authorities displayed remarkable tolerance by allowing her to continue her work as a Red Cross nurse.

Around this time, she wrote extensively for a few British newspapers and expressed her horror at the suffering she was witnessing in Brussels. Some of the sights she witnessed stretched her to the limit. As a Red Cross nurse, although she was critical of some of the actions of the German invaders, she managed to retain an outwardly neutral stance and was careful not to use any inflammatory language in her descriptions. Writing in *The Nursing Mirror and Midwives' Journal*, April 24, 1915, Edith Cavell described the situation in Belgium under German occupation. She wrote: "From the day of the occupation till now we have been cut off from the world outside. Newspapers were first censored, then suppressed, and are now printed under German auspices; all coming from abroad were for a time forbidden, and now none are allowed from England. The telephone service was taken over by the enemy, and we were shortly deprived of its use. The post, too, was stopped, and, though now resumed to certain towns and countries, all letters must be left open and contain no news of

---

[79] The Legend of Edith Cavell. Ranjit Jhuboo28 December 2018. AuthorHouse.

the war or of anything of importance. The few trains that run for passengers are in German hands, and wherever you go you must have, and pay for, a passport. No bicycles are allowed, and practically no motors (so the once busy and bustling streets are very quiet and silent?). So are the people, who were so gay and communicative in the summer. No one speaks to his neighbor in the tram, for he may be a spy. Besides, what news is there to tell, and who has the heart to gossip, and what fashions are there to speak of, and who ever goes to a concert or a theatre nowadays, and who would care to tell of their all-absorbing anxiety as to how to make both ends meet and spin out the last of the savings or to keep the little mouths at home filled, with the stranger close by? I am but a looker-on after all, for it is not my country whose soil is desecrated and whose sacred places are laid waste. I can only feel the deep and tender pity of the friend within the gates, and observe with sympathy and admiration the high courage and self-control of a people enduring a long and terrible agony. They have grown thin and silent with the fearful strain. They walk about the city shoulder to shoulder with the foe, and never see them or make a sign; only they leave the cafes which they frequent and turn their backs to them, and live a long way off and apart. A German officer on a tram politely asked a gentleman for a light; he handed him his cigar without a word, and, receiving it back, threw it in the gutter. Such incidents happen often, and are typical of the conduct of this much-tried nation."[80]

Belgium had little to thank the German invaders for. While most historians rightfully tend to focus on the numerous atrocities committed by German forces in World War II, not much attention is paid to the terrible acts of violence and destruction they perpetrated against the Belgian people in World War I, which can in many ways be regarded as a grim precursor. Many outside the country considered these acts as pure undiluted allied propaganda, but the truth was far more sinister. As the German juggernaut marched through neutral Belgium in 1914, it reduced once beautiful cities such as Louvain to rubble. They completely destroyed the world-famous library there that housed priceless,

---

[80] The Legend of Edith Cavell. By Ranjit Jhuboo (AuthorHouse, 2018).

centuries-old manuscripts. Then they conducted reprisals against the civilian population, summarily executing hundreds. Within two months of the occupation, it is estimated that the Germans murdered around five thousand five hundred Belgian citizens.

On August 15, 1914, two German battalions entered the town of Dinant. French soldiers successfully repulsed the first attack within a few hours. During this encounter a young French lieutenant by the name of Charles de Gaulle was wounded. Outraged at the show of defiance by the French army, the Germans made a second successful attempt to subjugate the town. In retribution against the citizens of Dinant, they executed 674 civilians, roughly 10 percent of the population. Among them were twenty-six pensioners, seventy-six women, and thirty-seven children. Félix Fivet, a three-week-old baby, was impaled on a German bayonet. More than 1,100 houses were completely destroyed, including the town hall and a museum. Eighty percent of the town was destroyed, and it was the largest massacre the Germans inflicted on the civilian population during that reign of terror in 1914. Those early British recruiting posters that depicted demonic German soldiers murdering babies and ravaging innocent women were dismissed as overzealous propaganda but were actually not all that far from the truth.

While attending her duties at the hospital, Cavell was introduced to two members of an old aristocratic family. Prince Reginald de Croÿ and his wife, Princess Marie, were to have a profound influence on her life. In the fall of 1914 two Belgian ladies, Henriette Moriame and Louise Thuliez, had been secretly tending wounded English soldiers since the fateful battle of Mons in August. They approached the Prince and Princess and asked them if they could assist in finding a way to help repatriate the unfortunate soldiers. A decision was taken to hide them at de Croÿs' home, Chateau Bellignies, near Mons where they would be provided with fake passports and a Belgian guide to help them on their way to safety. The secret password for the organization was "Yorc," the name of Croÿ in reverse.

The chateau soon became a safe haven for English and French soldiers seeking to escape across the border to the Netherlands and eventually back to England. Edith Cavell's Medical Institute became an integral part of this clandestine escape route. In the fall of 1914, two stranded British soldiers found their way to Nurse Cavell's Medical Institute where, regardless of the imminent danger, she hid them for two weeks. Others soon followed and every one of them was surreptitiously smuggled out to neutral territory in the Netherlands. Pt. Arthur Wood, one of the soldiers of the 1st Battalion, Norfolk Regiment, who'd fought at the Battle of Mons, recognized a print of Norwich Cathedral on the wall of Cavell's office. She still harbored great affection for her home county. She asked the soldier to take home her Bible and a letter for her mother.

Between November 1914 and July 1915, Cavell was instrumental in helping to organize the repatriation and escape of around two hundred people. In order to do this efficiently, she made contacts with various secret services and associations. She stayed at a café in Ghent, an important underground meeting place for the organization on several occasions. It was incredibly precarious work that demanded steel nerves and total dedication from all participants. She knew the incredible risk that she was taking, and was fully aware of the dire consequences if she was discovered, but this didn't deter her in the slightest. She regarded the concealment and repatriation of these men as a humanitarian act just as worthy as tending the sick and wounded. Ultimately fastidious and methodical in her work, the men who came to her were asked to sign papers giving their consent for a surgical operation. They were assigned fictitious illnesses, and their names, ages, dates of arrival and departure, and photos of them were all entered in a secret ledger. When the soldiers were spirited away, she would write to her mother describing the men who lodged with her and the guides who led them to safety. In these letters she would obliquely ask for news of their safe arrival in England on the premise that these some of the men were relatives of nurses in the School.

The network depended on everyone doing their part—but this was Belgium, a land with divided allegiances and double dealing, so something was going to give. Two of Cavell's colleagues noticed that she had become more withdrawn and less communicative but they had no idea why. Alongside the escape organization and the increasing difficulties in providing reliable guides and sufficient money for the escapes, her mentor Dr. Depage was busy working on the allied side of the war front and his wife Marie had left for America to raise money. Marie was drowned along with approximately 1,200 other passengers on the Lusitania when a German U-Boat torpedoed the ship on its voyage from America. At around the same time as Marie Depage's death, German Secret Police began to close in on the escape operations. Their purpose at this juncture was to gather information, but they didn't make any arrests until they could ascertain the full extent of the organization's operation and find out precisely who was involved. Cavell's status within the network had elevated and she had become a prime suspect, but there still wasn't enough evidence for the police to move in. She was becoming increasingly burdened with running the training school and supervising the building of the new school. She labored on in an atmosphere that was becoming increasingly charged with fear and suspicion. The net was closing.

Cavell's connection to Brussels native Philippe Baucq was widely known inside the organization. Baucq was an active member of the underground who played an important role in disseminating the clandestine newspaper *La Libre Belgique* (Free Belgium) and assisted in organizing the "Mot du Soldat," (the soldier's word), a service that provided a communication link between soldiers at the front and their relatives in occupied Belgium. He often worked as a guide, escorting escapees to the Dutch border.

Working in a Red Cross hospital demanded that wounded of all nations could be treated there indiscriminately, and Edith Cavell adhered stringently to this ruling. She had been warned by contacts that it was entirely possible that the German authorities were aware of her activities, but this didn't dissuade her from continuing her work. By the early summer of 1915, she was in imminent danger of being arrested. Most biographers believe the real villain in Cavell's story was Frenchman Gaston Quien, later convicted as a collaborator. She wouldn't have noticed that a certain wounded French soldier by the name of George Gaston Quien was a plant placed there by the German authorities. Quien had defected to the German side in exchange for his release. Disguised as an allied soldier in need of safe passage out of the country, he successfully infiltrated the network and passed on enough secret information to implicate Edith Cavell. Aware that the net was closing, she had taken precautions and secretly destroyed any incriminating documents she had in her possession. Precisely how much she knew about the information being carried on the bodies of the men she saved—written on cloth and sewn into clothes or hidden in shoes—remains quite a contentious issue to this day.

When Philippe Baucq was arrested in Brussels, a list containing Edith Cavell's name was found in his possession. The die was cast. She was promptly arrested and taken to Saint Gilles prison where she remained incarcerated for the next ten weeks, the last two of them in solitary confinement. Her small cell was sparsely furnished, containing a bed that folded to make a table, a small cupboard, and a washbasin. Her nurses sent flowers and she spent her time embroidering and reading her copy of the *Imitation of Christ* that had been sent to her by her friend Sister Wilkins.

Brand Whitlock wrote a letter to Baron von der Lancken, Chief of the Political Department of the German General Government in Belgium and German Military Governor Baron von Bissing dated October 11, 1915:

> *"Your Excellency,*
>
> *"I have just heard that Miss Cavell, a British subject, and consequently under the protection of my Legation, was this morning condemned to death by court-martial.*
>
> *"If my information is correct, the sentence in the present case is more severe than all the others that have been passed in similar cases which have been tried by the same court, and, without going into the reasons for such a drastic sentence, I feel that I have the right to appeal to his Excellency the Governor-General's feelings of humanity and generosity in Miss Cavell's favor, and to ask that the death penalty passed*

on Miss Cavell may be commuted, and that this unfortunate woman shall not be executed.

"Miss Cavell is the head of the Brussels Surgical Institute. She has spent her life in alleviating the sufferings of others, and her school has turned out many nurses who have watched at the bedside of the sick all the world over, in Germany as in Belgium.

"At the beginning of the war Miss Cavell bestowed her care as freely on the German soldiers as on others. Even in default of all other reasons, her career as a servant of humanity is such as to inspire the greatest sympathy and to call for pardon.

"If the information in my possession is correct, Miss Cavell, far from shielding herself, has, with commendable straightforwardness, admitted the truth of all the charges against her, and it is the very information which she herself has furnished, and which she alone was in a position to furnish, that has aggravated the severity of the sentence passed on her.

"It is then with confidence, and in the hope of its favorable reception, that I beg your Excellency to submit to the Governor-General my request for pardon on Miss Cavell's behalf."[81]

It was a poignant and passionate appeal that sadly fell on deaf ears. There was never any possibility of clemency or a reprieve. When the British Foreign Office decided to publicize letters and reports from

---

[81] Brand Whitlock, "Brand Whitlock's Letter to Baron von der Lancken," Edith Cavell 1865-1915 (September 9, 2015), https://edithcavell.org.uk/edith-cavells-life/account-by-reverend-h-stirling-gahan-on-the-execution-of-edith-cavell/brand-whitlocks-letter.

Brand Whitlock in *The Times*, the German authorities, and Baron von der Lancken in particular, were horrified. He immediately summoned Whitlock to his office on Monday, October 25, 1915, and demanded that the head of the American Legation make a formal apology. He told Brand Whitlock to his face that he, as Head of the American Legation, had openly lied about his frequent inquiries regarding Edith Cavell's condition and representation, and he insisted that the American Legation had never asked to be kept informed about the legal process.

Gaston de Leval claimed that he initially wanted to defend Edith Cavell in front of the German court martial, but for some inexplicable reason the German authorities flatly refused. Another Belgian lawyer, Sadi Kirschen, was appointed as the legal representative, but failed to have the death sentence commuted. Leval was later rightfully accused of not having done enough to save Cavell's life.

Initially denied visits or legal representation, September tenth, as previously mentioned Sadi Kirschen was appointed as her defense lawyer, but he wasn't allowed to visit her or to review the charges and was refused permission to view the trial documents. The specific charge against Cavell under paragraph sixty-eight of the German military penal code was "Conducting soldiers to the enemy." This was a lesser charge than "espionage," which carried a death sentence. When questioned she replied, "My preoccupation has not been to aid the enemy but to help the men who applied to me to reach the frontier. Once across the frontier they were free."[82] Technically she only helped these men get out of Brussels, and this fact should have figured in her trial. Aiding and abetting their escape would have been a less severe charge than the one she was facing. She never denied the charge, but it is widely known that she was a prolific correspondent, and the Germans were in possession of a letter that had been recently delivered to her through the American Legation. Even though she was clearly in possession of illegal correspondence, she was never accused of illegally sending or receiving mail. It's also alleged that she openly admitted to the charge against her to avoid being charged of

---

[82] Silent in an Evil Time: The Brave War of Edith Cavell. By Jack Batten (Tundra Publishing).

having conducted other seditious activities, which may have incriminated other conspirators. It was to be a closed trial, and neutral observers were not going to be allowed to attend.

Five German judges were appointed to try the case, but only the central prosecutor, military judge Eduard Stoebar, a man who had a dubious reputation was the only name known.

On October 7, 1915, Edith Cavell and other accomplices who worked for the escape network appeared before this military tribunal. The tribunal organized by the German military authorities took place in the Belgian Senate Chamber. Determined not to bring her profession into disrepute, Edith Cavell faced her accusers wearing civilian clothes. The trial of all the thirty-five accused took just two days. None of the accused were permitted or allowed decent legal representation. There was never any question of Edith being found not guilty. In her painfully honest way, she admitted culpability. The only question was the severity of the sentence the tribunal would impose. The harbinger of doom was the Military Governor of Brussels, General von Sauberzweig, a bitter and vengeful individual who bore a personal grudge against the British because his son had been blinded fighting them.

The British government appears to have remained discomfortingly inert throughout this whole process. Internal Foreign Office memos record one official assuring colleagues that Mr. Brand Whitlock "will see that she has a fair trial." Sir Horace Rowland, the FO's top official, agreed. "I am afraid we are powerless."[83] The sentiment was echoed by Lord Robert Cecil, who joined the coalition government in 1915 as an undersecretary for foreign affairs after working for the Red Cross. "Any representation by us," he advised, "will do her more harm than good." They appear to have abandoned Ms. Cavell to her fate, or maybe there was a more sinister reason for their lackluster approach?

None of the accused was present when October 11, 1915, the German judge passed sentence on Edith Cavell, Philippe Baucq, Louise Thulliez, a French teacher from Lille, Countess Jeanne de Belleville, and Louis

---

[83] Edith Cavell: Nurse, Martyr, Heroine. By Diana Souhami (Hachette).

Séverin, a Belgian pharmacist, were all condemned to death. Others who were arrested at the same time received varying prison sentences. At 8:30 p.m. on October eleventh, Edith Cavell was informed by the German Army Chaplain, Father Le Sueur, of her impending fate and that she had only a few hours left to live. Le Seur was able to arrange a visit by the Anglican Chaplain, Reverend H. Stirling Gahan. Reverend Gahan arrived at the St. Gilles prison at 10:00 p.m. Edith Cavell had unfolded her bed and was in her dressing gown. They talked and Edith Cavell said that after so many years of bustling activity, she regarded her solitude as cathartic.

Reverend Gahan had brought his Communion Set, so together they took the bread and wine and said the Blessing before speaking the words of the hymn: "Abide With Me." Gahan said to her before leaving that "We shall always remember you as a heroine and a martyr" to which she replied, "Don't think of me like that. Think of me as a nurse who tried to do her duty."[84]

Reverend Gahan wrote, "On Monday evening, October 11th, I was admitted by special passport from the German authorities to the prison of St. Gilles, where Miss Edith Cavell had been confined for ten weeks. The final sentence had been given early that afternoon.

"To my astonishment and relief I found my friend perfectly calm and resigned. But this could not lessen the tenderness and intensity of feeling on either part during that last interview of almost an hour. Her first words to me were upon a matter concerning herself personally, but the solemn asseveration which accompanied them was made expressly in the light of God and eternity.

"She then added that she wished all her friends to know that she willingly gave her life for her country, and said: 'I have no fear nor shrinking; I have seen death so often that it is not strange or fearful to me.'

"She further said, 'I thank God for this ten weeks' quiet before the end. 'Life has always been hurried and full of difficulty. This time of rest has been a great mercy.' 'They have all been very kind to me here. But

---

[84] Ibid.

this I would say, standing as I do in view of God and eternity, I realize that patriotism is not enough. I must have no hatred or bitterness towards any one.'

"We partook of the Holy Communion together, and she received the Gospel message of consolation with all her heart. At the close of the little service I began to repeat the words, 'Abide with me,' and she joined softly in the end.

"We sat quietly talking until it was time for me to go. She gave me parting messages for relations and friends. She spoke of her soul's needs at the moment and she received the assurance of God's Word as only the Christian can do. Then I said 'Good-by,' and she smiled and said, 'We shall meet again.'"[85]

Attempts to appeal for clemency were orchestrated by Hugh Gibson of the American Embassy (Brand Whitlock was ill), who enlisted the help of the Spanish Ambassador, the Marquis de Villalobar, and the Netherlands ambassador Maurits Van Vollenhoven. General von Sauberzweig had no intention of deviating from the sentence and informed Gibson the executions were scheduled to take place early on the following morning. The German authorities were hoping that her execution would just be a drop in the ocean; there was absolutely no chance of a reprieve.

Edith Cavell was executed by firing squad October 12, 1915. She is also often erroneously depicted wearing a nursing uniform when she was executed, but this was pure propaganda.

The final moments of her life were noted by Father Le Seur: "When we arrived at the Tir National, a company at full war strength (two hundred and fifty men) stood there, in accordance with the regulations, under the command of a staff-officer. A Military Court Councillor, Dr. Stoeber, with his secretary, Capt. Behrens, in command of St. Gilles prison, an officer from the Commander's office, and a medical man, Dr. Benn, were on the spot. We clergymen led the condemned persons to the front. The company presented their rifles, and the sentence was about to be read aloud in German and in French, when M. Baucq called out with a clear voice in French: 'Comrades, in the presence of death we are all comrades.' He was not allowed to say anything more. The sentence was read out, and then the clergymen were permitted to have a last word with the condemned persons. I thought I had to make this as brief as possible. I took Miss Cavell's hand and only said (of course in English) the words: 'The Grace of our Lord Jesus Christ and the love of God and the Communion of the Holy Ghost be with you for ever. Amen.' She pressed my hand in return, and answered in those words: 'Ask Mr. Gahan to tell my loved ones later on that my soul, as I believe, is safe, and that I am glad to die for my country.'

"Then I led her a few steps to the pole, to which she was loosely bound. A bandage was put over her eyes, which, as the soldier who put it on told me, were full of tears. Then a few seconds passed, which appeared to me like eternity, because the Catholic clergyman spoke somewhat longer with M. Baucq, until he also stood at his pole.

"Immediately the sharp commands were given, two salvoes crashed at the same time, each of eight men at a distance of six paces, and the two condemned persons sank to the ground without a sound. My eyes were fixed exclusively on Miss Cavell, and what they now saw was terrible. With a face streaming with blood, one shot had gone through her forehead, Miss Cavell had sunk down forwards, but three times she raised herself up without a sound, with her hands stretched upwards. I ran forward with the medical man, Dr. Benn, to her. He was doubtless right when he stated that these were only reflex movements."[86]

Edith Cavell was forty-nine years old. She remained magnanimous even when facing imminent death, forgiving her executioners, even willing to admit the justice of their sentence. Her last words according to Father Le Soeur were "*Ma conscience est tranquille Je meunt pour Dieu est ma Patrie.*" (My conscience is clear. I die for God and my country.) Stories circulated that the execution squad fired wide and that she fainted

---

[86] Edith Cavell: Nurse, Martyr, Heroine. By Diana Souhami (Hachette).

and was finally put to death by a German officer. This is pure conjecture because reliable witness accounts make no reference to this at all. Across the British Empire her death was used to galvanize public opinion against the Germans. It's maybe cynical, but probably true to suggest that Nurse Edith Cavell was worth more to the British dead than alive. In Britain, recruitment numbers rose from five thousand to ten thousand a week following her execution. The frenzy of outrage and condemnation that it provoked around the world was unprecedented. Recently uncovered evidence suggests that she may indeed have worked as a spy, moreover further British documents indicate that the German authorities acted in accordance with the law when they sentenced her death. Edith Cavell deserves to be remembered as a hero even if she was a spy.

Some say that legendary French singer Edith Piaf was named after her.

CHAPTER THIRTEEN

From Here to Hemingway

During the greater part of World War I from July 20, 1914, until November 9, 1917, General Cadorna was the Italian army's chief of staff. He was eventually relieved of command for his alleged role in Italy's resounding defeat at the epic Battle of Caporetto. Cadorna allegedly executed more of his own men than all the other incumbent armies together. Between 1915 and 1917, more than half a million Italian soldiers met violent deaths on what was known as the "Isonzo Front." Hundreds of thousands more succumbed to disease, hunger, freezing temperatures, and avalanches. Hemingway vividly referred to the aftermath of the Battle of Caporetto in his famed novel *A Farewell to Arms*, but he wasn't actually there at the time.

On April 6, 1917, the United States declared war on Germany. That day, the American Red Cross (ARC) renounced its neutrality and assumed its other federally-chartered military role to provide medical assistance to the country's armed forces in wartime. It looked good on paper, but in reality, just like the U.S. armed forces, the organization was drastically ill prepared for the role it was assuming. It's entirely possible that Hemingway saw the ARC has a possible vehicle to get to the front faster than the army. Six base hospitals had already been dispatched to support the British Expeditionary Force in May 1917. Most, if not all, of these Red Cross hospitals were already operating as American-sponsored independent institutions even before America's entry into the war. The first of these to be appropriated by the Army and ARC was the "American Ambulance in Paris." The order came directly from Major General "Black Jack" John J. Pershing, commander of the American Expeditionary Force.

In 1917 a young man from Illinois called Ernest Miller Hemingway left his job at the Kansas City Star newspaper, and signed on as an ambulance driver with the American Red Cross. He was eighteen, eager for action and adventure and responding to a recent recruitment drive. He had attempted to enlist in the army, but had been rejected due to poor vision, undeterred he would get to the front. Many believe that Hemingway harbored a pure undiluted determination to join the fray and get stuck in, but this wasn't the case at all. As far as he was concerned the location of the front was superfluous, the fight was on and he wanted to get close (but despite his pugnacious attitude to just about everything he didn't want to get *too* close). In desperation to join up in some form or another, he had even written to his sister explaining that he was planning to join the Canadian army. He settled for the National Guard but soon discovered that they had no intention whatsoever of getting sent overseas. Hemingway was bitterly disappointed.

According to one version of Ernest Hemingway's account, one day a wire service story came to the telegraph desk, dealing with the Red Cross's need for volunteers to work with the Italian Army; being the impetuous young man that he was, he cabled his application before the paper even had a chance to publish the item. This was a barometer of how eager he was for adventure. He was no different from countless other young men who had signed up, fired with patriotic zeal, and testosterone fueled temporary insanity and determined to "do their bit."

In 1917 the Italian Army had suffered a crushing defeat inflicted by the Austro-Hungarian and German forces at a place called Caporetto. Italian army casualties were unprecedented, and estimated to have numbered been between 700,000 and 750,000. During the final three months of 1917, the enemy had taken 335,000 prisoners, including those belonging to labor battalions and those hospitalized soldiers left to their fate as the Italian army retreated. Austro-Hungarian troops occupied two thousand square miles of Italian soil and had requisitioned an innumerable amount of Italian Army supplies. The aspirations of the Central Powers to neutralize Italy and take it out of the war completely had almost succeeded.

Austro Hungarian and German forces had achieved a resounding victory, which had shaken allied confidence. The situation was approaching its nadir and questions were being asked at allied command as to whether the Italian army would be able to recover. While Italian forces were regrouping and replacing men and equipment lost at Caporetto, U.S. Captain George Utassy, who had been recently appointed administrative officer at Italian field headquarters in charge of all ambulance units in Italy, issued a strong appeal stating that "one hundred Americans were needed at once by the American Red Cross for ambulance service behind the Italian lines." The wording of the article was unambiguous:

"It is a splendid opportunity for men of independent means, over draft age, who are strong and healthy and able to drive automobiles. Consideration will be given to men 25 years or over, who are exempt for minor defects. All cost of equipment and living expenses abroad will be covered by the American Red Cross, and transportation expenses will be paid, if necessary."[87]

The eventual response was overwhelming and resulted in a veritable flood of aspiring applicants. Young Hemingway saw this as his ticket, his opportunity, and he wasn't going to let it slip. He had heard and even possibly read, the rousing sermons of Dr. William Barton of the First Congregational Church, encouraging America's young men to go to war, but these didn't necessarily inspire Hemingway's burgeoning sense of adventurism. The sister of this minister was Clara Barton, the woman who had originally founded the Red Cross in America.

---

[87] The Letters of Ernest Hemingway: Volume 1: 1907-1922 (Cambridge University Press, 2011).

Once Hemingway's application had been approved, he managed to fit in one last fishing trip before boarding a train in Kansas May 12, 1918, to go to New York and join the Red Cross. When the train pulled into the Grand Central Terminal in Manhattan, he had roughly ten days to acclimate to his new role as a Red Cross volunteer before boarding the steamship that would take him overseas. His initiation into the Red Cross in New York coincided with a peak of support for the beleaguered Italians as they anticipated further enemy offensives that summer. While Hemingway was in New York, Mayor John F. Hylan announced the opening of "Red Cross Week" scheduled to start May twentieth. Two days previous to the commencement of various Red Cross fund raising and PR activities, thousands of war workers had paraded through Manhattan amid a milling throng of spectators. Hemingway, who hadn't yet fired a shot in anger or touched foot on foreign soil, had no problem participating in the parade. Unencumbered by not having actually done anything useful for the Red Cross, he even wrote a letter home about the attention he and his organization received during the pageant. "We paraded 85 blocks down 5th Ave today and were reviewed by President Wilson. About 75,000 were in line and we were the star attraction."[88] A few days later, May twenty-third, after a few minor delays, he was aboard the steamship Chicago heading to Bordeaux. He wasn't very complimentary about the vessel he was sailing on and described it as "the rottenest tub in the world." It was a relatively uneventful crossing of the Atlantic, because by that time in 1918 the danger of being attacked by a German U boat was highly unlikely. This fact appears to have disappointed Ernest somewhat, because in his anticipation of partaking in some action, he had strolled the decks each day hoping to spot a U boat, and by the time the ship docked in Bordeaux on June first, he felt that he'd been defrauded.

Thanks to seemingly endless alcohol fueled poker games and shooting craps, the one thing he did achieve during the voyage was making new friends. Seemingly endless alcohol fueled poker games and shooting

---

[88] Idem

craps helped him interact with his shipmates and establish firm friendships. This was more in tune with the developing character of Ernest Hemingway. The esprit de corps that he established with two of these men endured through his service until well after the Great War had ended.

A few days after his arrival on the French mainland he was on a train heading to Paris. He appears to have been completely captivated and enthralled by European culture and that first visit to Paris would initiate a love affair with the city that would endure for decades. He quickly registered at "Nr 4 Place de la Concord," the Red Cross headquarters in Paris. It was a luxurious former palace complete with ornate crystal chandeliers, red carpets, and high ceilings that must have seriously impressed the naïve young man from Kansas, unaccustomed to such luxury and comfort. He wasn't given any immediate tasks so those first days could be donated to pure hedonistic pursuits, such as getting to know the city and checking out all the major attractions.

While he was there the Germans lobbed over some high velocity shells fired from their feared "Big Bertha" from seventy-one miles away. The first attack occurred on Good Friday in 1918 and continued thereafter. The gun was capable of firing a 234 lb. shell to a range of around eighty miles. A total of around 320 to 367 shells were fired at a maximum rate of roughly twenty per day. The shells killed 250 people, wounded 620, and caused considerable damage to property. The name Big Bertha was applied, incorrectly, by members of the Allied forces to these extreme long-range cannons that were better known simply as the "Paris Guns." Blasé Parisians were generally unfazed by these regular bombardments and went about their lives, business as usual. This appears to have inspired the thrill-seeking Ernest, who actually hired taxis so he could go and inspect the shell craters made by these big guns.

He left Paris on an overnight train that arrived in Milan on Friday, June seventh. As soon as he got there, he was exposed to the to the brutal reality of war when an explosion occurred in a storage area at a nearby munitions factory. Hemingway and his colleagues were transported to the site to assist in collecting dead bodies and other remains that littered the countryside. This wasn't the front line and most of the victims were women, but it would have been a gruesome introduction nonetheless. Two days later he was finally where he wanted to be, in proximity to the front lines. The Red Cross post at Schio had thirty Red Cross ambulance drivers and was located at the base of the Little Dolomites four miles, give or take, from the Austrian positions. It was nowhere near the Piave River where some of the most intense action developed during June and July of that year.

Hemingway and authority were not a particularly great combination and he complained vociferously about his Captain there from day one. Captain Bates was a veteran of many great WWI battles. He was a strict disciplinarian who valued his role supervising the drivers and managing the vehicles. He often conducted personal reconnaissance of the front in preparation for major offensives and made frequent visits to check the conduct of his volunteers. His insistence on exemplary behavior by his personnel at all times didn't endear him to them. By the same token, Hemingway wasn't all that popular with some of his fellow volunteers either, who criticized his impatience to experience front line action. Devoid of any serious activity and a pool of eighteen pairs of drivers operating in shifts lasting two or three days, it is unlikely that he would have been called upon to sit behind the steering wheel of an ambulance other than to pose for a photograph. Consequently, he set the parameters for his future image, passing his time drinking copious amounts of alcohol, gambling, fighting, and attempting to impress some of the local ladies. Light duties, inertia, and a pool of eighteen pairs of drivers operating in shifts lasting two or three days, it is unlikely that Ernest would have been called upon to sit behind the steering wheel of an ambulance other than to pose for a photograph.

The Austrians launched a major offensive June 15, 1918, with a massive but predicted bombardment, and once the fighting kicked in it didn't engage the services of Ernest's "Section 4" unit in Schio. He supplemented some of his time writing flippant articles for the Section 4 self-printed monthly magazine called *Ciao*, but things were about to change. On June twenty-fourth, he was finally presented with an opportunity to participate in some action but it wouldn't have much to do with driving an ambulance. Volunteers were requested to staff canteens in proximity to the front lines, and hormonally-challenged Hemingway immediately took one step forward. He joined a unit that reached forward areas using kitchens mounted on wheels that became known as "rolling kitchens." It sounded like a good idea at the time, but it didn't take long before Ernest began complaining that he should be driving an ambulance instead of dispensing cigarettes and chocolate.

At least now he had the chance to see some battle conditions up close. When he arrived at the most active combat zone along that front, the Austrians had already been defeated in the Battle of the Piave, and the Italians were in the midst of launching their counterattack. As the Austrians retreated he travelled on some of the same roads and finally got to satiate his thirst by witnessing scenes of terrible carnage and devastation. Shortly after this he would experience a little more than he had bargained for when he was severely wounded. He had succeeded in getting closer to the action and was incongruously using a bicycle to distribute his supplies of tobacco and confectionery to front line Italian troops at a place called Fossalta.

Suddenly an enemy trench mortar shell exploded nearby, showering shrapnel into Hemingway and three Italian soldiers. One of whom was killed outright, another severely wounded while Hemingway absorbed hundreds of pieces of metal into his legs, scrotum, and lower abdomen. Despite his horrific wounds he displayed remarkable endurance and courage by carrying one of the wounded soldiers fifty yards before he was hit in the leg by machine gun fire. Even this didn't knock him off his feet; he somehow managed to move a further hundred yards before he blacked out. It was a tremendous display of resilience in terrifying conditions. Apart from the physical wounds that he sustained, the event left an indelible stain on his mind that would remain with him for the rest of his natural life. It wouldn't, however, deter him from seeking other wars, other battles and other conflicts.

During his subsequent six months of convalescence, he fell head over heels in love with an American Red Cross nurse, Agnes von Kurowsky. He would recount the incident and transpose versions of his experiences through his literary classic such as *A Farewell to Arms*. Agnes von Kurowsky was twenty-six and Hemingway was eighteen when they first met and the age difference clearly featured in their brief relationship. She was the inspiration for the character of Catherine Barkley, the tragic heroine of *A Farewell to Arms*. Agnes did not reciprocate his passion, and five months after their first meeting she flatly rejected his marriage proposal. Their love affair came to an abrupt end when Hemingway returned to the U.S. and she unceremoniously dumped him for an Italian officer.

Many years later he recounted some of his experiences in *Men at War*, a compilation of eighty-two prominent short historical war stories from around the world. He wrote, "When you go to war as a boy you have a great illusion of immortality. Other people get killed not you. Then when you are badly wounded the first time you lose that illusion and you know it can happen to you. After being severely wounded two weeks before my nineteenth birthday I had a bad time until I figured out that nothing could happen to me that had not happened to all men before me. Whatever I had to do men had always done. If they had done it then I could do it too and the best thing was not to worry about it."[89]

It's entirely possible that due to his service with the National Guard he could have eventually been selected for the regular army despite his problematic eyesight, but the Red Cross was a more immediate solution for one so impatient. He was, however, one of the first Americans to receive a commendation in World War I when the Italian government presented him with the Silver Medal of Valour. He had earned it and he deserved it. He went on to write various literary masterpieces. He took his own life in July 2, 1961, in Ketchum, Idaho. He was Ernest Hemingway.

---

[89] Men at War. Various Authors including Ernest Hemingway, Leo Tolstoy, Winston Churchill (CreateSpace Independent Publishing Platform, 2015).

CHAPTER FOURTEEN

American WWI Nurses

The Army Nurse Corps was founded in 1901 and was initially comprised of around over one hundred female nurses, but they were not given appropriate titles, military status, or even uniforms. When the armistice was declared 21,000 women had either served in France or at home as members of the Army Nurse Corps. It was the illustrious actions of these women that helped to expand the Nursing Corps, which inevitably led to the development of an early rank structure, as well as a system to allocate money for retirement.

During World War I (WWI), the U.S. Army assigned nonphysicians to front line trenches for the treatment of casualties. These men would treat soldiers directly at the site of injury if casualty levels were light. Otherwise, company litter bearers would carry the injured to company aid stations and then to battalion aid posts. Treatment included hemorrhage control and the splinting of fractures. At the company aid station, medical personnel would further control hemorrhage, adjust bandages and splints, and administer anti-tetanus serum before moving the injured to the battalion aid post. From there, the wounded were evacuated to ambulance dressing stations at the point nearest the front lines that ambulances could reach safely. At these stations, battlefield placement of dressings and splints could be revised if necessary, and the wounded were triaged for further transport. Procedures developed and implemented in WWI would also be used in WWII.

Mrs. Mary Borden-Turner was the founder of Mobile Surgical Hospital No 1. She was an American woman married to a British Army officer. Her hospital was established in the French section on the Western Front and she recorded her experiences for posterity. She wasn't particularly impressed with two American Red Cross ambulance men. As they arrived, she was dealing with an abdominal injury. She said, "When the surgeon came he said impatiently. Ah a serious wound, he should be hastened to the rear at once". The surgeon tried to unbutton the soldier's soaking trousers, but the man gave a scream of pain. "For the sake of God, cut them. Do not economize".[90]

An assistant (with heavy, blunt scissors) half cut, half tore the trousers from the man who screamed in agony as clots of black blood rolled from the wound, then a stream bright and scarlet, which was stopped by a handful of white gauze, retained by tightly wrapped bands. Then the surgeon shot a stream of morphine into the wounded man's leg. Two ambulance men came in—Americans in khaki who were ruddy, well-fed, careless. They lifted the stretcher quickly, skillfully. The wounded soldier opened his angry eyes and fixed them furiously. "Bloody foreigners" he screamed. "What are you here for? To see me, with my bowels running out on the ground? Why didn't you come for me ten hours ago, when I needed you?"

They shoved him into the ambulance, buckling down the brown canvas curtains by the light of a lantern. One cranked the motor, then both clambered to the seat in front, laughing. They drove swiftly but carefully through the darkness, carrying no lights. Inside, the man continued his imprecations, but they could not hear him.

In a field hospital, some ten kilometers behind the lines, one soldier lay dying. For three days he had been dying and it was disturbing to the

---

[90] The Backwash of War. Ellen N.LaMotte.

other patients. The stench of his wounds filled the air, his curses filled the ward. For he knew that he was dying and that he had nothing to fear. He gave forth freely to the ward his philosophy of life, his hard, bare, ugly life, as he had lived it, and his comments on patriotism, as he understood it. For three days, night and day, he screamed in his delirium, and no one paid much attention. The other patients were sometimes diverted and amused, sometimes exceedingly annoyed, according to whether or not they were sleepy or suffering. And all the while the wound in the soldier's abdomen gave forth a terrible stench, filling the ward, for he had gas gangrene, the odor of which is abominable. In the bed next to him lay a man with a fecal fistula, which smelled atrociously. The man with the fistula, however, had got used to himself, so he complained mightily. On the other side lay a man who had been shot through the bladder, and the smell of urine was heavy in the air round about. Yet this man had also got used to himself, and he too complained about the awful smell of gas gangrene, and gangrene is death, and it was the smell of death that the others complained of. Two beds farther down, lay a boy of twenty, who had been shot through the liver. Also his hand had been amputated, and for this reason he was to receive the Croix de Guerre.

One woman who experienced the American WWI effort was Alice L. Mikel Duffield. Part of the U.S. Army Nurse Corps, she was based in Fort Pike, Arkansas. She wrote: "War broke out, I think it was April, and I was still in training. And it had been raining, but it cleared off. It was warm, even then. [My] mother had a baby boy, born on my birthday, when I was twenty years old, and I didn't even see him, 'cause I wasn't there. But later, he got sick, and Mama wrote to me and she said, "Alice, I am just worn out. Your little brother has pneumonia, that's what Dr. Means says. And I take care of him, day and night, and try to do the cooking, and everything else to keep the household running. If you could just get off for a short time and help me till I get rested, I surely would appreciate it." And Miss Tye said, "There's no reason why you can't go." She said, "What do you know about pneumonia?" I said, "Nothing." We had one man that had pneumonia. Now, we had people, doctors, lecturing on all these subjects. We got all our schoolbooks given [to us]; we didn't pay for them, they were given to us. And different things about different diseases. All of them, free. We got notebooks, pencils, everything furnished. Three meals a day, and a place to sleep. And our laundry was done. And that's the only way we could have [done] it.

"Giving baths to the boys, took their temperatures. I don't remember giving any medicines. You see, the office there were so many nurses there they gave those girls the medicines, to the older nurses, they gave the medicines. And, we took their temperatures. And we were told… they didn't put the thermometers in their mouths because they ran high temperatures, and people with high temperatures would bite the thermometers, so we put them under their arms, and held their arms down."[91]

Those Red Cross nurses who served on the Western Front in World War I were quick to improvise when the first deadly clouds of gas floated toward the allied positions on March 10, 1915, at Ypres, Belgium. The Germans flagrantly discharged 168 tons of chlorine gas from strategically placed cylinders. The deathly cloud drifted toward Allied trenches, inflicting over 5,000 casualties. In the absence of respirators, the nurses drenched their sanitary towels in eau de cologne and held them over their faces and those of the wounded soldiers.

These incredibly brave women were volunteers; they went wherever they were sent, were present in all the theatres of war, and in many cases faced similar dangers to those of the soldiers in or near the frontlines. Most volunteer nurses worked in one of the Casualty Clearing Stations (CCS), usually a safe distance from the front, and normally comprised of large tents some containing up to eight hundred beds. A typical CCS could hold up to 1,000 casualties at any time, and would normally admit fifteen to three hundred cases, in rotation. At peak times of battle, even the CCS's often became inundated with casualties. Serious operations such as limb amputations were carried out here. Some CCS's were specialist units designated for nervous disorders, skin diseases, infectious diseases, certain types of wounds, and much more. They didn't move location very often, and the transport infrastructure of railways usually

---

[91] Lost Voices: The Untold Stories of America's World War I Veterans and their Families. By Martin King and Michael Colins (Roman and Littlefield, 2018).

dictated their location. Most evacuated casualties came away from the CCS by rail, although motor ambulances and canal barges also transported casualties to Base Hospitals, or directly to a port of embarkation. The term shell shock is most readily associated with World War I but scant attention was paid to those who exhibited symptoms of this condition. The original assumption was that being too close to an exploding shell had the potential to cause dysfunctional behaviors. Nevertheless, a soldier displaying neuropsychiatric symptoms yet showing no physical signs could errantly be accused of cowardice and in the case of the British and French armies they could even be sentenced to death as a warning to other so called "malingerers." The British used the acronym LMF on the papers of shellshock cases. It meant "Lacking Moral Fiber."

The Great War saw many notable innovations such as the introduction of blood banks, mobile X-rays, aerial photography, and the inclusion of women in uniform. It was during the war that sanitary napkins for women were first invented. When America officially entered the Great War, Kimberly-Clark started to mass-produce the padding for the purpose of using it for surgical dressing. Red Cross nurses assigned in the battlefields discovered that this product was remarkably absorbent, so they decided to use it for their own personal hygiene; hence, this seemingly innocent item brought great fortune to the once-small firm. Kimberly-Clark's new invention of sanitary napkins was branded Kotex, which stood for "cotton texture." They became available to the general public in October of 1920, only two short years after the Armistice was signed.

During the cataclysmic Champagne-Marne Operation that began on July 15, 1918, there was a mobile hospital unit precariously close to the front line.

Captain Fordyce St. John Commander of Mobile Hospital No. 2 wrote: "During the first two hours of the barrage, the shells were landing approximately 125 yards beyond us and causing no trouble but at about six in the morning the enemy changed his range and the shells began dropping short and long, the typical range-finding method used, and it was now impossible for the wounded to reach us. This situation continued until seven o'clock, when high explosives began falling among the thin wooden sheds of the hospital itself, so that it became necessary to issue an order to evacuate the wards and to remove all patients to the underground dugout. Before this could be accomplished, the shock ward was pretty well demolished by two direct hits. Several casualties had already occurred, and, before the shacks could be evacuated, two more men were killed, one of whom was decapitated. A Presbyterian Hospital nurse in charge of this ward was dragged protesting from her post forty seconds before the shell hit the frail building. Patients were being killed as they were unloaded from ambulances. Some ten minutes later another shell demolished the corridor connecting the operating shack with the wards and one wall of the operating room was badly splintered. As it was becoming apparent that it was impractical to carry on, orders were given to cease operating and all personnel were ordered to the dugout after the last patient had been placed there."[92]

They were lifesavers and the angels of mercy who paid the ultimate price on many occasions. More often than not their deeds would be forgotten, cast aside while others reaped the credit for a battle won or a successful assault on enemy positions.

Another American nurse Julia C. Stimson directed the activities of ten thousand Army nurses during the final days of the war, and through the difficult post-war demobilization period. Thanks to her dedication and her efforts, thousands of wounded soldiers received good medical care. For her service in France during the war, the United States government awarded Stimson the Distinguished Service Medal. Other nations bestowed the British Royal Red Cross, First Class; the French *Medaille de la Reconnaissance Francaise*; the *Medaille d'Honneur de l'Hygiene Publique*; and the International Red Cross Florence Nightingale Medal. After the war she continued to work as a nurse and was a key recruiter of female nurses in WWII.

---

[92] Neighbors, 1892-1967: A History of the Department of Nursing, Faculty of Medicine, Columbia University, 1937-1967, and Its Predecessor, the School of Nursing of the Presbyterian Hospital, New York, 1892-1937. By Eleanor Lee (Columbia University-Presbyterian Hospital School of Nursing Alumnae Assn., 1967).

Among other things the Great War went a long way to redefining class restrictions on both sides of the Atlantic, which had up until 1917 prevented privileged young women from even considering the prospect of employment in the nursing profession. Patriotism was a great leveller. One socialite named Winifred Tittman, the daughter of a prominent St. Louis family, recalled a half century later, "Once my brother was shot down, I was allowed to go to nursing school."[93] Army nurses were presented with military medals for bravery and some even died for their country, but they were not granted actual military rank until 1920. Even then, the conferred title didn't allow them the same privileges as commissioned ranks.

When America entered the war in April 1917, the army's need for nurses was so desperate that a voluntary aide system was even considered. Despite the army's aspiration to enroll more nurses, military authorities didn't provide them with the same benefits afforded to other branches even when they were discharged from service. On top of this, the pecuniary dissimilarities between serving men and women only served to reinforce Julia Stimson's feminist ideologies.

Another notable WWI nurse that pre-empted American involvement was Isabel Anderson.[94] She was the wife of U.S. Ambassador Larz Anderson who was the American envoy to Belgium from 1911 to 1912. When the call came, she was one of the thousands of women who volunteered to help in the war effort. At home in the U.S., she raised funds for war related charities before volunteering to work for the American Red Cross in field hospitals directly behind the front lines. She remained there for eight months. For her service she was awarded the French *Croix de Guerre* and the Belgian Queen Elisabeth Medal for her work. In her book *Zigzagging* she relates some of her experiences as a front-line nurse. Her experience living as the wife of a U.S. Ambassador in Brussels had

---

[93] Gateway Heritage: Quarterly Journal of the Missouri Historical Society-St. Louis, Missouri, Volumes 20-21 Missouri Historical Society (1999).

[94] Easing Pain on the Western Front: American Nurses of the Great War and the Birth of Modern Nursing Practice. By Paul E. Stepansky (MacFarland).

provided Isabel with a decent knowledge of the French language, and this proved to be an advantage when she was at the front.

She frequently uses the names and phrases in her descriptions: "The hospital buildings looked like a cross be-tween racing-stables on a track and a Japanese Shinto temple, with a slight resemblance to a lagging camp. In other words, many long, low, unpainted barracks, with small cloth windows.

"My first day, a handsome man with thick black hair and big black eyes was brought in right from the trenches. He had both legs cut off, but fortunately, he did not know it. I stayed by his bedside most of the time after he came out of the ether, but he died at ten that night. I became especially interested the next day in a little blond man who had been wounded three times and given every kind of decoration. He died that evening. After this I was so exhausted and sad that I hardly slept, and cried most of the night. Then I caught cold in my side, and blistered it with iodine. Indeed, I was discouraged, but kept going and didn't lose an hour's work.

"In the ward we gave salt injections and morphine shots, etc., and had blood transfusions. I mixed every known kind of drink, and fetched and carried, and made bandages de corps, and covered rubber rings, for most of the wounded had to sit on them in bed, and every night rubbed down a dozen men with alcohol and powder. Of course there was a grandfather on our ward. One always called the older ones grandfather (grandpere) or my oldie (mon vieux). Our grandfather was only thirty years old, though he had a beard and looked almost any age. He was nicknamed 'The Tiger,' and was certainly a rough customer. His arm and leg on one side were both badly wounded, and he had a hole in his forehead besides. A Carrel tube is-sued from his bandaged head, and I was obliged to squirt Dakin solution into it every two hours. He called the tube his telephone and used to tell me what he heard through it. We couldn't make out if he was a little out of his mind or very original and amusing."

American nurse Ellen La Motte[95] also volunteered to serve close to the front lines in Europe. From the outset she was determined to work as a nurse and she satiated this ambition years before the United States entered the war. She had started her nursing career as a tuberculosis nurse in Baltimore, Maryland. On arriving in Europe, she first went to the American Hospital at Neuilly, a French commune just west of Paris, only to discover to her chagrin that it already had more than enough volunteers. She was then introduced to Mary Borden, the daughter of a wealthy American businessman and wife of an English merchant, who was running a field hospital in Belgium. La Motte joined her and served in a French field hospital with the French Army from 1915 to 1916. By 1915 she was in Belgium. Her 1916 book *The Backwash of War* was one of the first publications to present international audiences with firsthand views of the day-to-day horrors she witnessed. The book was considered so explicit at the time that it wasn't reprinted until 1934. In one chapter titled *Locomotor ataxia*, which means loss of coordination of movement, Ellen described her experiences:

"The seriously wounded were unloaded carefully and placed upon beds covered with rubber sheeting, and clean sacking, which protected the thin mattresses from blood. The patients were afterwards covered with red blankets, and stone hot water bottles were also given them, sometimes. But in the sorting tent there were no such comforts. They were not needed. The sick men and the slightly wounded could sit very well on the backless benches till the Medecin Major (doctor in charge) had time to come and examine them.

"Quite a company of 'sitters' were assembled here one morning, helped out of two big ambulances that drove in within ten minutes of each other. They were a dejected lot, and they stumbled into the tent unsteadily, groping towards the benches, upon which they tried to pose their weary, old, fevered bodies in comfortable attitudes. And as it couldn't be done, there was a continual shifting movement, and unrest. Heavy legs in heavy wet boots were shoved stiffly forward, then dragged

---

[95] The Backwash of War: The Human Wreckage of the Battlefield as Witnessed by an American Hospital Nurse. By Ellen Newbold La Motte (2019).

back again. Old, thin bodies bent forward, twisted sideways, coarse, filthy hands hung supine between spread knees, and then again the hands would change, and support whiskered, discouraged faces. They were all uncouth, grotesque, dejected, and they smelt abominably, these poilus (hairy), these hairy, unkempt soldiers. At their feet, their sacks lay, bulging with their few possessions. They hadn't much, but all they had lay there, at their feet. Old brown canvas sacks, bulging, muddy, worn, worn-out, like their owners. Tied on the outside were water cans, and extra boots, and bayonets, and inside were socks and writing paper and photographs of ugly wives. Therefore the ungainly sacks were precious, and they hugged them with their tired feet, afraid that they might lose them.

"Then finally the Major arrived, and began the business of sorting them. He was brisk and alert, and he called them one by one to stand before him. They shuffled up to his little table, wavering, deprecating, humble, and answered his brief impatient questions. And on the spot he made snap diagnoses, such as rheumatism, bronchitis, kicked by a horse, knocked down by dispatch rider, dysentery, and so on a paltry, stupid lot of ailments and minor accidents, demanding a few days, treatment. It was a dull service, this medical service, yet one had to be always on guard against contagion, so the service was a responsible one. There is much bronchitis in Flanders, in the trenches, because of the incessant Belgian rain. They are sick with it too, poor devils. So said the Major to himself as he made his rounds."[96]

The advent of World War I saw spectacular advances in anesthetics, aseptic surgery, and bacteriology, as well as the growth of the civilian and military medical professions. By the end of the war infection rates were down to 0.1 percent. One in five of the American troops who fought the Spanish in 1898 contracted typhoid, but very few did in 1917–1918. Diseases ranging from syphilis to "trench foot" (a condition similar to frostbite caused by feet being constantly immersed in water) did not threaten the belligerent armies' fighting strength and efficiency. This was largely due to the rise of a professional medical corps before 1914, as well

---

[96] *The Backwash of War: The Human Wreckage of the Battlefield as Witnessed by an American Hospital Nurse.* By Ellen Newbold La Motte (2019).

as new developments in preventive medicine. These afflictions affected proportionately fewer than in previous wars, and most of those who did fall victim could return to active duty.

Still more remarkable was medicine's success in rehabilitating the wounded, and this more than anything else accounted for the armies' ability to keep fighting despite frequently appalling casualties. When the casualties of the Great War returned home many were psychologically damaged. They would rarely (if ever) relate their experiences. These silent ones were not the same men who had rallied to the various flags of belligerent nations in 1914 and in 1917. Their pain was deep, profound and in many cases enduring. Then there were the ones with horrific facial damage. Reconstructive surgery was still in its infancy so many were reduced to wearing prosthetic facial features, noses, eyes, chins and sometimes whole jaw bones. Estimates vary, but at least 12 percent of all men wounded suffered from facial injuries, and roughly one-third of these were permanently disfigured. The road to recovery for these men was often fraught with terrible pain and anguish.

These were the ones for whom the war never ended; most wars rarely do. If the prospect of being blown to smithereens wasn't bad enough, in 1918 there was another ominous prospect looming on the horizon, which wouldn't be discriminate as a German shell or bullet. Some "experts" have made comparisons between the 2020 pandemic and the so-called "Spanish Flu," but there are marked differences. The devastating Spanish Flu that eventually overwhelmed almost every corner of the world began in 1918. Granted there are some vague similarities, but in all fairness Spanish Flu makes COVID-19 pale by comparison. Back then approximately one-third of the planet's population became infected, and it is estimated that Spanish Flu killed an estimated twenty million to fifty million victims, including some 675,000 Americans. Spanish Flu was an H1N1 virus with genes of avian origin, but so far there is no universal consensus regarding where the virus originated. At the time of writing this, there have been roughly 581,000 COVID-19 related deaths in the U.S. Though the number of worldwide deaths is much less than 20 to

50 million, American deaths are comparable to those inflicted by the Spanish Flu.

As far as the United States is concerned, Spanish Flu first reared its ugly head in the U.S. on March 4, 1918, at Fort Riley in North Central Kansas on the Kansas River. It was a military training facility housing twenty-six thousand aspiring "Doughboys." When Army cook Albert Gitchell from Haskell County, reported sick there was audible cheering from the barracks, but not for long. Within days, 522 men at the camp had also contracted the virus, but Chef Albert was the first recorded victim. He reported sick and was shown to have a fever of 103. Then Corporal Lee Drake arrived displaying almost identical symptoms. One by one, men with fevers of 104 degrees Fahrenheit, pallid complexions, and horrendous, hacking coughs made their way to the infirmary. The first serious flu pandemic had arrived. By the way, Albert survived. He died in 1968 at the age of seventy-eight.

There is vociferous disagreement regarding the origins of the disease. Some even claim that it began in the U.S. while others refer to newly unearthed records claiming that, as with COVID-19, China may have been the source of the pandemic. That said, it's popular to blame China for everything at the moment up to and including indigestion. It's true that ninety-six thousand Chinese laborers were mobilized and set to work behind the British and French lines on World War I's Western Front. These laborers referred to by some as "Coolies" repaired tanks, assembled shells, transported supplies and munitions, and dug allied trenches. They literally reshaped the war's battle sites but never participated in the combat. This flu then spread throughout France and hitched a lift with the AEF (American Expeditionary Force) and other military forces as they journeyed back to their respective countries. There are many theories, but that's all they are, simply "theories."

The world's populations have endured and survived pandemics before. Take the, "Bring out your dead, Black Death" that consumed Europe in 1347 and claimed two hundred million lives in just four years. "Lockdown" isn't a new concept, either. By the early 1500s, England introduced the first laws intended to separate and isolate the sick. Homes stricken by plague were marked with a bale of hay strung to a pole outside. If you had infected family members, you had to carry a white pole when you went out in public. That would definitely have encouraged "social distancing."

Nineteen-eighteen was a seminal year in the history of World War I. When peace broke out with the armistice that signaled the end to all hostilities November 11, 1918, some places along the Western front in Europe were destroyed to such an extent that local engineers required maps from the town hall vaults to identify the exact locations of certain villages and hamlets. So why "Spanish Flu" if it didn't originate in Spain? During World War I, Spain remained neutral and had ample time to deal with the disease and its terrible consequences, which included claiming the name, although why the Spanish would want to be literally associated with a deadly pandemic remains a mystery as perplexing as bullfighting. The problem was that the international community erroneously assumed that the disease emanated from Spain, but even so-called "experts" can get it wrong, and frequently do.

CHAPTER FIFTEEN

U.S. Medics in World War II

The legacy of experience gained from previous wars paved the way for a new generation of talented medical personnel in World War Two. When America joined in World War Two. The overall effectiveness of combat medics and military personnel providing front line trauma care increased significantly thanks to medical innovations.

It was a war waiting to happen because during the years that followed the Great War, Hitler managed to completely refute the punitive conditions imposed by the inevitably flawed "Treaty of Versailles" and annex all the territories that had been previously requisitioned from Germany. By 1940 Japan had officially recognized the leadership of Germany and Italy and the new order in Europe when it signed a document known as the "Three-Power Pact." The three countries agreed to co-operate and assist one another with all political, economic and available military means.

The real game changer occurred on December 7, 1941, when Japan bombed Pearl Harbor and Germany declared war on America. Meanwhile in Washington, D.C., it was generally acknowledged that reorganization within the U.S. Army was long overdue. When Germany had invaded Poland in 1939 the U.S. Army was ranked in strength only seventeenth in the world, marginally behind Romania. At that time there were only three effective divisions within the whole United States. It's remarkable to reflect that only six years later they would number over six million personnel. With a new war came new advances in medical innovation.

When German biochemist Gerhard Johannes Paul Domagk (1895–1964) published his findings in 1935, doctors discovered that one of his compounds called Prontosil reduced many bacterial infections. Subsequently, other researchers developed derivatives based on the Prontosil sulfonamide group. The resulting so-called sulfa drugs revolutionized medicine and became particularly popular during WWII.

The discovery of Sulfanilamide significantly reduced the mortality rate during World War II. Sulfa drugs were used routinely to control such diseases as pneumonia, gonorrhea, meningitis, dysentery, and streptococcal infections. American soldiers were taught to sprinkle sulfa powder immediately on any open wound to prevent infection. Every soldier was issued a first aid pouch that attached to his or her waist belt. The first aid pouch contained a package of sulfa powder and a bandage to dress the wound.

In 1928, Scottish bacteriologist Sir Alexander Fleming initiated a series of experiments that involved the common staphylococcal bacteria. He had begun his work during the Great War when he began experimenting with antibacterial substances. In 1921 he discovered lysozyme, an antibiotic enzyme that attacks many types of bacteria. A few years later in 1928 he noticed that an uncovered Petri dish sitting next to an open window had become contaminated with mold spores. Fleming observed that the bacteria in proximity to the mold colonies were dying off. Proof of this was the dissolving and clearing of the surrounding agar gel. He managed to isolate the mold and identify it as a member of the Penicillium genus.

Later on, Fleming discovered that this residue was particularly effective against all Gram-positive pathogens, which are responsible for diseases such as scarlet fever, pneumonia, gonorrhea, meningitis, and diphtheria. He discerned that it was not the mold itself but the residue it had produced that had eliminated the bacteria. Consequently, he named it the "mold juice" penicillin. The potential medicinal value of this discovery would have wide ranging consequences. He immediately understood the potential medical value, but it wasn't a done deal. Fleming had neither the resources nor the means to manufacture enough penicillin to be useful in practice; however, his discovery was dismissed as no more than a laboratory curiosity. A further ten years would pass before a team of scientists at Oxford University rediscovered Fleming's work. By this time, they had more convincing evidence of the remarkable powers of penicillin. The timing was bad because by then Britain was heavily involved in WWII and unable to provide the necessary funds to develop the drug further. This prompted the team to seek help in the United States.

In 1941 John Davenport and Gordon Cragwall,[97] two representatives from the pharmaceutical company Pfizer, attended a symposium. During the symposium researchers from Columbia University presented irrefutable evidence that penicillin could effectively treat infections. These two men recognized the potential and promptly offered Pfizer's assistance. It would take another couple of years and involve many pitfalls before they could effectively mass-produce what became widely regarded as the world's first "wonder drug."

By June 1942, only enough penicillin had been produced to treat ten men. Army trials of the drug began in spring 1943 and were so successful that when Pfizer demonstrated that its scientists had found a deep tank fermentation process to produce the drug, the government purchased twenty-one billion units. Eventually Pfizer produced 90 percent of the penicillin that landed with Allied forces at Normandy on D-Day in 1944 and more than half of all the penicillin used by the Allies for the remainder of the war. It helped to save countless lives. Penicillin remains one of the most active and safe antibacterial available. Further medical innovations such as blood plasm, and whole blood also helped to reduce the fatality rate of battle casualties. WWII marked a watershed in the history of vaccine development as the military, in collaboration with academia and industry, achieved unprecedented levels of innovation in response to war-enhanced disease threats such as influenza and pneumococcal

---

[97] Blind Quest: Deceived by Experience. By Bert Tucker Jr. (iUniverse).

pneumonia. Wartime sponsored government programs contributed to the development of new or significantly improved vaccines that tackled ten of the twenty-eighth vaccine preventable diseases identified in the 20th century. It's somehow ironic that over seventy-five years later, Oxford University scientists working with AstraZeneca were among the first to develop the first vaccinations to prevent the spread of COVID-19. Pfizer was also successful in trialing and bringing their own version vaccine to the market.

By 1943 in the United States, the demand for trained nurses reached beyond previously accepted racial barriers. When the Cadet Nurse Corps was established in that year both black and white women, along with a few Native American women, entered the nursing profession. There were even a few Japanese American internees in the program. Over 115,000 Cadets were enrolled in both federal and non-federal hospitals. When General James Carre Magee was appointed Surgeon General on June 1, 1939, he and his staff went on to play an integral part in the introduction of new drugs for military use and insisted on immunizing every soldier against typhoid and paratyphoid fevers, smallpox, and tetanus, which kept the incidence of these diseases so low as to be almost insignificant. By the end of 1942, he had thirty thousand doctors and twenty thousand nurses serving the military.

Nurse Dorothy Barre served in the U.S. Army in World War II. (She first appeared in the book *Voices of the Bulge*, published by Zenith Press in 2011.) She enlisted in the Army July 5, 1943, as a Registered Nurse (serial number N- 752 051) and was stationed at Camp Edwards on Cape Cod before being assigned to the 16th General Hospital, which was re-organized at Fort Andrews, Massachusetts, on September 1, 1942. On August 25, 1943, the unit was moved to Fort Devens, where the nurses went through Basic Training.

On December 28, 1943, the "Hospital" with one hundred nurses, five hundred corpsmen and support staff, sixty male officers and four Red Cross volunteers embarked on the transport ship Edmund B. Alexander that was anchored in Boston Harbour. The ship departed on December 29, 1943, and arrived in Liverpool England January 8, 1944. Then the

16th General Hospital set up at Oulton Park, Cheshire, England, on January 8, 1944, before being moved to Penley Hall Flintshire, in Wales.

On August 13, 1944, the 16th General Hospital arrived at Southampton Docks and boarded the Dutch ship Nieuw Holland' at 1:00 p.m. before being shipped across the English Channel. They arrived at Utah Beach, Normandy, France via LCT's at 7:00 p.m. The 16th General Hospital was dispatched to a bivouac area near Enghien-les-Bains, France, roughly ten miles from Paris on October 2, 1944, where it remained until October 9, 1944. Then it was relocated to Liege, Belgium on October 11, 1944. Dorothy later recalled, "We were a complete unit with casts, dental equipment, X-ray machines, surgical equipment, everything. They put us in tents in a field in Normandy for six weeks, then sent us to Paris, then Liege, Belgium. I worked as a nurse in the surgical orthopedic wards. We were set up in Liege before the Bulge broke, and we were in tents that would hold thirty patients at a time. In the center of each tent was a potbelly stove that kept us warm, and we had surgical carts we could use for dressings. When the Bulge broke, Liege was an ammunition dump, so they were sending buzz bombs toward the city. We were in that alley of buzz bombs, and when we heard them, a patient would run out and see what route they were on. There were three routes that they fired over us. Over that period, we were hit three times with the buzz bombs, not where the patients were. We did not have any casualties. We were ten or twelve miles from the fighting. But one time one of the buzz bombs hit nearby, one of the houses, and we admitted Belgian patients. I had a mother and a daughter, and the daughter died. The doctor and I worked together to help them until they could get the mother to the Belgian hospital in Liege.

"Before the Bulge, we treated soldiers sometimes, but when the Bulge started, we got them from army trucks or stretchers. They might just be wrapped in blankets, the young fellas, and we got them washed up. Sometimes we would have four nurses to one guy, getting them washed up, pajamas on, their dressings checked. We would ask them if they had pain, and we carried codeine and aspirin in our pockets. I remember sitting on the cots and talking with the guys. They would always ask me where I came from, since I have a Boston accent. Sometimes they would stay with us for just eight or ten hours. "The patients would get a good meal and cleaned up and given penicillin too. After they were well enough, they were flown to Paris or London. We had a few specifically from the 101st paratroopers and engineers as well. I think we knew that the Germans had broken through and the Bulge was getting close to us. We didn't go into the city, about four miles away. We stayed in a chateau, a stone building. I was on the third floor, and there were seven to eight nurses to a room with a potbelly stove in the center. We had showers down in the cellar. Some nights, some of us would go down in the cellar because of those buzz bombs. They would start them about eleven o'clock at night and go until about two or three in the morning, and then they would start again at four in the morning."[98]

All allied soldiers in WWII received fairly frequent medical check-ups. Ensuring that a soldier was fit and healthy enough to perform his or her duties was just as important as tending the wounded. One soldier, Major Earl Edwards was preparing to take 2nd Battalion, 22nd Infantry, 4th Infantry Division ashore on D-Day (June 6, 1944). But before he could begin his assault into France, Edwards had a certain problem he had to deal with. A few days before the actual landing he was suffering from a debilitating case of hemorrhoids that was causing him considerable discomfort. He found his ailment even affected his gait. He asked his roommate to report his condition to the Colonel. He was sure his medical situation would prevent him from making the landings. In his memoirs Edwards described the events: "Later in the day an ambulance drove up to our quarters and two medics came in and said that I was to come with them. They helped me to the ambulance where I found Col. Tribolet and the Regimental Surgeon, Dr. Kirtley. We drove away and soon parked in front of a U.S. Field Hospital. Col. Tribolet and Dr. Kirtley went in and soon returned. We then drove awhile and parked in front of another hospital.

---

[98]   Voices of the Bulge: Untold Stories from Veterans of the Battle of the Bulge. By Michael Collins (Martin King. Voyageur Press, 2011).

"The same thing happened. So we drove on to another. This time some medics came out and carried me in and within a short time I was operated on. After an hour or so of recovery I was carried back to the ambulance, which returned me to my quarters, and I was placed again on my bunk. All this time no explanations whatever. I later learned that Col. Tribolet was determined that I would command the 2nd Battalion in the invasion so he and Doc Kirtley decided to take me to a hospital and ask if they would operate on me and immediately release me to their care. If the answer was 'no' they simply carried me to another hospital and so on until one agreed.

"So I went into the landings with a large wad of cotton taped to my rear. Fortunately, the salt water and a few artillery rounds cured me. I don't remember ever thinking about it after we landed."[99]

Despite advances in psychiatry, it appeared that in WWII the lessons of WWI had been largely ignored. There was still a stigma attached to those diagnosed with shell shock or combat fatigue. On April 26, 1943, General Omar N. Bradley issued a directive, which established a holding period of seven days for psychiatric patients at the 9th Evacuation Hospital, and for the first time the term "exhaustion" was prescribed as the initial diagnosis for all combat psychiatric cases. Another reason exhaustion was chosen was because it was considered to have no negative connotations that could relate it to the actual problem of neuropsychiatric disturbance. The implication being that psychiatric breakdown was the result of natural fatigue, and that simple rest was sufficient to return men to duty. In World War II, combat stress casualties accounted for between 20 to 30 percent of those wounded in action. In August 1943 Lieutenant General George S. Patton visited a hospital near Palermo. His well-publicized berating of a psychiatric casualty caused a media frenzy and a public outcry, but it also highlighted the issue of combat exhaustion and provided the necessary stimulus the military needed to deal this debilitating condition.

---

[99] To War with the 4th: A Century of Frontline Combat with the U.S. 4th Infantry Division, from the Argonne to the Ardennes to Afghanistan. By Martin King, Jason Nulton, and Mike Collins (Casemate, 2016).

Apart from a glaring lack of knowledge concerning psychiatric problems that could arise from exposure to combat, the U.S. military had to deal with other pressing issues exacerbated by antiquated thinking. There was still racial segregation in the U.S. armed forces at that time, and during World War II the U.S. Army Nurse Corps was initially reluctant to accept black nurses into the service on the premise that assignments available to black nurses were limited, because they were only allowed to care for black troops in black wards or hospitals. In January 1941, the U.S. Army established a quota of fifty-six black nurses for admission to the Army Nurse Corps. Through the efforts of the National Association of Coloured Graduate Nurses (NACGN), the Army quota was abolished before the end of the war, consequently black women served with distinction in various capacities. When the war ended in September 1945 just 479 black nurses were serving in a corps of fifty thousand, because a quota system imposed by the segregated Army during the last two years of the war restricted the number of black enrollments. By late July 1945, there were 512 black women in the Army's Nurse Corps, including nine captains and 115 first lieutenants. Of the three units that served overseas, one was a group of sixty-three black nurses who worked with the 168th Station Hospital in Manchester, England, caring for wounded German prisoners. In 1943, for example, the Army limited the number of black nurses in the Nurse Corps to 160.

In December 1941, just a few days after the bombing of Pearl Harbor that initiated America's entry into World War II, a Detroit mother named Sylvia Tucker visited her local Red Cross donor center to donate blood. She had been inspired by the rousing calls on national radio and wanted to do her part. When she arrived at the center, the supervisor promptly turned her away and refused to accept her donation. Orders from the National Offices prohibited African American blood donors at this time. Mrs. Tucker was so shocked by the incident that she wrote an articulate and emotional letter of protest to first lady Eleanor Roosevelt.

"I was shocked and grieved to learn that the 'eternal color question' was paramount to the grave war situation. After

explaining that both my loyalty to my country and to my young son, who will be eligible for Military Service in two months, prompted my offer, I challenged the doctor to accept my blood and place it in a container and label it 'Negro Blood' and after due process make it available for some Negro mother's son, who, like his white American brothers-in-arms, most face shot and shell and death as these things know no 'color line.' I begged him to do this, I would have paid for the processing, if need be. I fear that the time may come when all blood white or black may be needed, so many, many lives depend upon it! This is not a letter of hate, despite the disappointment and bitter-ness and humiliation I suffered at the Red Cross on last Thursday rather, it is an appeal for immediate mutual understanding and good-will and the exercise of 'the brotherhood of God and the fellow-ship of Man.' The American Red Cross holds the destiny of thousands of human being[s], white and black, make them understand that 'We are Americans, too,' and we want to make the blood sacrifice we must make the blood sacrifice not only for the present '5%' but for the vast percentage of soldiers that must be called and must face the Hell of War before this conflict is over."[100]

Charles R. Drew was an African American physician who had developed ways to process and store blood plasma in "blood banks" and conducted pioneering research on typing, preserving, and storing blood for later transfusion. In 1941 he became the first African American surgeon selected to serve as an examiner on the American Board of Surgery. He was later appointed director of the first American Red Cross Plasma Bank. Late in 1941, the surgeons general of the United States Army and Navy took the ignominious decision to inform the Red Cross that only blood from white donors would be accepted for military use. Despite the fact that it had been conclusively proven that there were no racial

---

[100] One Blood: The Death and Resurrection of Charles R. Drew. By Spencie Love.

differences in blood, the military was conceding to prevailing social bias and substantial political pressure.

In January 1942, the War Department revised its position, agreeing to accept blood from black donors, but rigidly insisted on adherence to segregation of the blood supply. A black soldier could receive a blood transfusion from a Caucasian donor if there was nothing else available but the reverse wasn't possible. Surprisingly enough the esteemed Red Cross not only accepted that decision but also declared that it had no interest in meddling with social/racial controversies. Red Cross officials later offered that those who persisted in criticizing the policy were unpatriotically attempting to cripple the blood donor service and thus harm the war effort itself.

Drew openly denounced the policy, stating that there was absolutely no scientific evidence of any difference based on race, and declared that the racial segregation of blood was in contravention to scientific fact, and an insult to patriotic black Americans. Due to this he was asked to resign from the Red Cross. He returned to Washington, D.C., and became the head of Howard University's Department of Surgery and later Chief Surgeon at the University's Freedman's Hospital. Drew died on April 1, 1950, in Burlington, North Carolina, from injuries sustained in a car accident while en route to a conference at the Tuskegee Institute in Alabama. The government rescinded its policy on blood segregation eight months after Drew's death.

Della H. Raney, a graduate of the Lincoln Hospital School of Nursing in Durham, North Carolina, was the first African American nurse to be commissioned as a lieutenant in the Army Nurse Corps during World War II. Her first tour of duty was at Fort Bragg, North Carolina. As a lieutenant serving at the famous Tuskegee Army Airfield in Alabama, she was appointed Chief Nurse, Army Nurse Corps in 1942, effectively the first African American to receive this appointment. She later served as Chief Nurse at Fort Huachuca, Arizona. Raney was promoted to captain in 1945. After the war, she was assigned to head the nursing staff at the station hospital at Camp Beale, California. In 1946, she was promoted to major and served a tour of duty in Japan. Major Raney retired in 1978.

The remarkable Mabel Staupers had championed Raney's cause. During World War II, Ms. Staupers worked as the Executive Secretary of the National Association of Colored Graduate Nurses (NACGN) where she led the movement to gain full integration of Black nurses into the armed forces and the professional nursing organizations. The purpose of the NACGN was to confront the marginalization of black nurses and to advance the standing and best interests of trained nurses. The organization accomplished higher standards of nursing and an overall shift in society by exposing the burdens of discrimination and segregation. The struggle to achieve recognition, status, and acceptance of Black nurses into the institutional structures of American nursing was significantly advanced because of her leadership.

Mabel Staupers was born in Barbados, West Indies, on February 27, 1890. In April 1903 her family migrated to the United States and in September of that year settled in Harlem, New York. After early education in New York, she was admitted to the Freedmen's Hospital School of Nursing in 1914. She completed the three-year course in 1917 and graduated with honors. In the same year she married Dr. James Max Keaton of Asheville, North Carolina. This marriage ended in divorce. In 1931 she married Mr. Frisby Staupers of New York City.

Her professional career began with private duty nursing in New York City and Washington, D.C. In 1920, in cooperation with the late Dr. Louis T. Wright and Dr. James Wilson, she organized the Booker T. Washington Sanatorium, the first facility in the Harlem area where Negro doctors could treat their patients. She served this institution as administrator and director of nurses. In 1921 she was awarded a working fellowship to the Henry Phipps Institute for Tuberculosis in Philadelphia, Pennsylvania. She was later assigned to the chest department of the Jefferson Hospital Medical College in Philadelphia. Her experience there with segregation and discrimination of staff and patients was one of the motivating forces that made her, in later years (again in cooperation with Dr. Wright), work for full and equal opportunity in all health programs and services and on professional nursing organizations in New York City and the Nation. She strove for the inclusion of Black nurses to the Army and Navy during World War II. African American nurses had shown interest in joining the Army Nurse Corps as early as 1927, to no avail. When a black nurse applied for admission to the Corps in late September 1940, she was told in no uncertain terms Army regulations made no provision for the appointment of Negro nurses. In 1940, when approached on the subject of using black nurses, Surgeon General of the U.S. Army Medical Corps James C. Magee had been non-committal is his response: "Their employment has been found impracticable in time of peace. You may rest assured that when military conditions make it practicable for the war department to use colored nurses they will not be overlooked."[101]

The American Red Cross, National Association of Colored Graduate Nurses (NACGN), and other nursing organizations protested the Army's policy of excluding African-American nurses. Ms. Staupers confronted President Franklin Roosevelt on the issue. Roosevelt responded by reassuring her that the War Department was considering the employment of black nurses. By April 1941 there were forty-eight Black nurses assigned to Camp Livingston, Louisiana and in Fort Bragg, North Carolina. The number of black nurses tripled by May of 1943.

During World War II, African American nurses served in all theatres of the war including Africa, Burma, Australia, and England. The first black medical unit to deploy overseas was the 25th Station Hospital Unit, which contained thirty nurses. The unit went to Liberia in 1943 to care for U.S. troops protecting strategic airfields and rubber plantations. The nurses wore helmets and carried full packs containing gas masks and canteen belts. The Red Cross arm bands and lack of weapons distinguished them from those who were actually fighting troops. Mabel Staupers continued to fight for the full inclusion of nurses of all races and this was finally granted in 1945. By the end of World War II, approximately six hundred African American nurses had served their country, and by 1948 the American Nursing Association allowed them to join their ranks.

Women Army nurses who served in combat areas during World War II were a vital element, but despite their massive contribution they

---

[101] The History of the U.S. Army Medical Service Corps. By Richard V. N. Ginn.

remained largely unrecognized for their service. One particular Black lady who volunteered to serve with a U.S. Army medical unit remained anonymous for over sixty-five years.

War and conflict can produce the most unlikely heroes and heroines. Augusta Chiwy was one such heroine. She died on July 23, 2015, at the grand age of ninety-four while living in a geriatric care home on the outskirts of Brussels and was buried in Bastogne with full military honors. Her character appeared all too briefly in the famed *Band of Brothers* series portrayed as "Anna from the Congo" in the *Bastogne* episode.

Augusta's story is quintessentially about two people: a doctor and a nurse whose paths would've never crossed had it not been for the siege of Bastogne. They had a relationship that left no time for romantic interludes. They were too preoccupied trying to save lives and care for wounded soldiers with little more than bandages and antiseptic powder, performing surgery with no surgical instruments and only Cognac for anesthesia.

In 1930 at the tender age of nine, Augusta was brought to Belgium by her white European father, a travelling veterinarian called Henry Chiwy. She was one of many mixed-race children who were becoming so ubiquitous in Congo that the Belgian government of the day had to enact a parliamentary motion to bring these children to Belgium. Augusta spent the remainder of her childhood in Bastogne, ultimately leaving for the northern Flemish town of Leuven in her early twenties to attend nursing school. After graduating as a fully qualified nurse, she remained in Leuven and worked at the Saint Elizabeth Hospital, which was staffed by the Augustine Congregation Sisters of Louvain. While there in December 1944, she decided to accept an invitation from her father to go home to Bastogne and spend Christmas with him and his sister-in-law (whom she called "Mama Caroline"). By December 1944 the allies had breached the Siegfried line in some places and were preparing to push the Nazis back beyond their own western border. Augusta's timing was atrocious. On the very day that she decided to make the trek to Bastogne three German armies launched a concerted offensive against thinly held allied positions in the Belgian Ardennes.

During the very darkest days of the Battle of the Bulge in World War II, she volunteered to work with the 10th Armored Division and then the 101st Airborne. Many, many Americans lived to tell the tale because of her. After WWII she didn't return to full time nursing until 1967. The reason was because Augusta suffered from a form of PTSD known as "Selective Mutism." Any mention of the war or Bastogne would make her clam up completely.

The surgeon at the 20th AIB Aide Station in Bastogne where Augusta worked was Dr. John "Jack" Prior who hailed from a small town in Vermont. Jack and Augusta weren't just from different countries with different languages. They were from different worlds. It was the fortunes of war that brought them together and tore them apart. But in the few weeks that they worked side by side in the Army hospitals, they forged a deep bond that endured for decades after the war.

On the morning of December 16, 1944, Augusta left Louvain by tram. When she reached Brussels to transfer southward, she discovered that all trains bound for Bastogne and Luxembourg were terminating at the city of Namur. From there passengers were loaded onto cattle trucks, the only form of transportation available and taken a further twenty miles to the town of Marche. It was a chilly ride. With temperatures plunging to minus twenty degrees Fahrenheit and colder, that December was the coldest winter in Northern Europe in living memory. After spending more than fifteen hours on the road and having used trains, trucks, a U.S. Army Willys Jeep, and even a bicycle, she finally reached Bastogne at around 11:00 p.m. that evening.

The town of Bastogne was no stranger to conflict. A group of devoutly religious nuns known as The Sisters of Notre Dame who ran Augusta's former school began preparing the cellars just as they had done in 1940. As worried Bastogne civilians began to flock there, Augusta volunteered to assist.

She was completely oblivious to the fact that three German armies had broken through the lightly defended western front in an all-out effort to seize the Port of Antwerp, with the intent of dividing the allies and ending the war. As they advanced westward, leaving a trail of destruction in their wake a significant "bulge" in the allied battle lines began to take shape, hence the name of this infamous battle. As the situation grew more desperate, the 10th Armored rushed three teams to Bastogne that constituted just 2,700 men. Among them with "Team Desobry" was Army Doctor (Captain) Jack Prior who found himself just north of Bastogne in the village of Noville attempting to hold back the enemy onslaught. Dense Ardennes mist exacerbated an already desperate situation, and after little less than forty-eight hours the diminutive force was overwhelmed and evacuated to Bastogne.

A few days later the strategically important market town of Bastogne became completely surrounded by enemy forces. After having lost a number of his men in Noville, Jack instructed his second in command Captain Irving Lee Naftulin to comb the market town for anyone with medical experience to aid their efforts. Naftulin found two people, a young nurse named Renee Lemaire, and Augusta Chiwy. Both women agreed to join forces with Jack to prepare and treat the steadily increasing number of casualties as U.S. forces struggled to maintain their tenuous hold on the city against repeated onslaughts by well-equipped German divisions. As German artillery fire began to intermittently fall inside the American perimeter, the small group set up shop in a recently abandoned building that had served as a grocery store. With living quarters upstairs and a cellar below, it was about the best location available for a new aid station.

Jack discovered that Augusta was incredibly adept at handling the bloodiest and most grave of injuries, handling amputees, bleeding, large thoracic wounds, and other results of battlefield trauma. Renee was the comforter—best at soothing soldiers in pain and keeping them clean. Because racism was still fairly institutionalized in the United States in 1944, Augusta, a mixed-race woman, was the subject of bigotry on more than a few occasions. There were many American soldiers who refused to be treated by her, to which Jack's response was usually, "She treats you, or you die." Augusta quickly discovered that death is a great leveler.

On a few occasions, Jack and Augusta made extremely risky trips to the front lines to evacuate the wounded. One of the most significant of these was at a promontory just outside Bastogne called Mardasson Hill, which today is the location of the largest American monument outside the United States. Here, Augusta and Jack came under intense rifle, machine gun, and artillery fire in a dangerously exposed position, but despite this they still managed to treat and evacuate several critically wounded men. Augusta, who wore a long nurses' gabardine, came through unscathed, but discovered several bullet holes in the garment. In later years, Augusta recalled in interviews that Jack had remarked, "Looks like they almost got you. It's a good thing you're small." She retorted that, "A black face in all this snow is an easy target. The Germans are just bad shots."

As the Nazi vice tightened its grip on Bastogne, casualties mounted considerably. And due to the intense, all pervading mist the Air Forces were unable to resupply the besieged garrison until December twenty-third. Up until that point Jack's medics were forced to use bed sheets and any other available fabric as bandages. In one extreme case, Jack and Augusta were forced to amputate one man's hand and leg using nothing more than the serrated edge of an Army issue survival knife and anesthesia provided by a bottle of requisitioned Five Star cognac.

On Christmas Eve, Jack and Augusta briefly left the aid station to enjoy a glass of champagne provided by a resourceful GI in the house adjacent. Once inside they heard the unmistakable drone of approaching aircraft, but what they thought was another airdrop was in fact an enemy bombing mission. Their aid station took a direct hit from a five-hundred-pound bomb. The percussion threw Jack to the ground and blew Augusta clean through a brick wall. Miraculously they both survived relatively unscathed, but their Aide Station was leveled to the ground, killing thirty patients inside along with the other Bastogne volunteer Nurse Renee Lemaire, whose fragile body was blown into two pieces. The following day Jack reported for duty at the 101st Airborne HQ at the Heintz barracks, and Augusta followed him.

They continued to work together almost ceaselessly day and night. They saved lives together and watched life slip away together. And on more than one occasion, they had barely escaped death together. Bastogne was liberated by General George Patton's 3rd Army on December twenty-sixth, and on January seventeenth, Jack and Augusta were forced to make their goodbyes. They wouldn't see each other again until more than five decades later. Their story is one of incredible bravery, compassion, and devotion. It's a story of tenderness in the midst of appalling inhumanity enriched with a depth of caring that went mostly unexpressed and unacknowledged.[102]

Jack returned home in 1945, became a respected pathologist, and raised a family. Augusta also survived to raise a family, but suffered severe post-traumatic stress for the rest of her life. In 1948 the Red Cross sent her a desultory letter of thanks for her service, but her incredible efforts were largely forgotten after the war—and she had absolutely no desire to recount them. After a fervent campaign to get Augusta the recognition she so richly deserved was launched in 2011, Belgian King Albert II officially declared her a Knight of the Order of the Crown, which is basically the equivalent of a knighthood. Then the 101st Airborne Division presented her with the Civilian Humanitarian Medal. Augusta had finally gotten her just acknowledgement.

Army Nurse Corps Veteran Isabelle Cook. Isabelle served during World War II. She had just graduated from Mount Sinai Hospital School of Nursing when the war broke out. Unbeknown to her family she volunteered to go oversees with the Army Nurse Corps. On May 5, 1943, Isabelle and her colleagues arrived in Casablanca, Morocco, and spent three months waiting for the Germans to be defeated in Tunisia. Over the next three years, the 3rd General Hospital would follow the front into Italy and then France. Cook celebrated the end of the war by marching in the VE (Victory in Europe) Day parade in Aix-en-Provence, France alongside Allied soldiers. The order came to close down the 3rd General in August 1945. She received her formal discharge in December 1945, having earned the rank of First Lieutenant.

She wrote a book about her experiences titled *In Times of War*. The following abridged interview was made for the Library of Congress Veterans History Project: "I didn't tell my family. I had a mother that

---

[102] Searching for Augusta – The Forgotten Angel of Bastogne. By Martin King (Lyonpress, 2019).

was a widow with five children and I didn't tell her. I didn't ask her permission, I just signed right up. And then waited impatiently for them to call me for the Service. Finally, in September of 1942, I got the call, proceed immediately to Camp Rucker, Alabama. Now, you can imagine the culture shock going from Manhattan down to Camp Rucker, Alabama in Ozark. And it was a tiny town of about 500 people, real southerners, and here are these northern Yankees that came to invade the area. And we had our basic training there and you could imagine civilians undergoing this basic training when we marched and had backpacks and everything else and all the soldiers in the camp lined up to see the nurses marching by and mis-marching, most of the time.

"But we made it through basic training. It was about six months. And then we got the orders to go overseas. And we ended back up in New York at the port of embarkation and we stayed there, processed, we were given all the clothes that we needed for overseas service.

"We were given permission to actually go home for one day to see the family. Mother was in shock when she knew that I was going overseas, but I had to make her understand that I felt it was my duty to be part of the Army. My brother was drafted and he was in the Army at the time. He went to Officer's Training School and he became an officer. He went -- we went on a troop ship that was SS Louis Pasteur. Originally, it was a French Army overseas for a luxury liner and they converted it into a troop ship and it was manned by British soldiers to transport American troops. Since it was a very fast ship, we just zigzagged right across the Atlantic. We didn't go in a convoy. We didn't know our final destination. This is in May 5th, 1943, but we ended up in Casablanca.

"We spent about three months in Casablanca because of the fact that the Germans were still fighting in Tunisia and our hospital, the thousand-bed general hospital was supposed to be set up in Mateur. That was just outside of Tunis. When the Germans were defeated in North Africa, then we got our orders to proceed to Mateur in Tunisia. I was one of the ten nurses that was chosen to go on the advance party. We travelled 1500 miles across country, across North Africa in a two and a half-ton truck, an open truck and the heat was -- in May was unbearable.

But we managed to go across. We slept in pup tents at night. We had the K-rations for food, but one night we actually spent in the -- the French Foreign Legion. We spent one night with them and we got a real hot meal and a bed to sleep in which was just wonderful.

"One night, we were able to go to a portable shower unit for the soldiers, for the combat soldiers, and they stopped the soldiers from going in to allow the ten nurses to take a shower, which was wonderful after two days being on the road. And, of course, we had the soldiers all lined up ready to wash our backs and do everything else. They were very helpful but, of course, I do think there might have been a hole in the tent but we never did find out for sure whether there was one or not.

"We finally arrived in Mateur. It had been bombed out and people were living in caves. And I asked the charge nurse, what was my duties as one of the ten people for setting up the hospital in Mateur and she said you'll be the housekeeper. Here I am about 22 years old, never took care of a house in my life and suddenly I'm the housekeeper. She said you'll be in charge of the laundry and the housekeeping duties. Well, I thought I don't know anything about it, but like Scarlett O'Hara, I'll worry about it when the time comes. But she said well, you can probably get the townspeople to do the laundry. Well, there was no town. It had all been bombed out and people were living in caves. So we took over the French Army barracks that were used as a hospital by the Germans.

"In fact, there were still German prisoners well they were German soldiers that were so severely wounded they could not be evacuated. They left one German doctor to care for them. So they immediately became prisoners of war. So we took care of them. There were German signs all over the place. Well, the rest of our unit arrived about several days later. They had had a terrible experience going cross-country in a -- in cattle cars and even one of our nurses had died as a result of heat -- the heat was so terrible.

"Well, we set up our entire hospital in about eight days, 800 tons of equipment, generators, we had our own portable generators and the whole hospital was set up and the nurses and the nursing personnel had tents. There were five of us in each tent and outside latrines and outside wash stations and things like that. The heat -- the -- we were getting the winds, the 'taraka' winds from the Sahara and living in the tents, it was pretty bad. But we were taking care of the casualties from Sicily. The Sicilian campaign had started and within about five days after we set up the hospital, we started receiving patients.

"They were evacuated by air and we acted as an evacuation hospital instead of a general hospital which takes care of the more severely wounded and those that needed to stay much longer. But we received about 2,000 patients. And as a result, we had to open another thousand-bed hospital on -- in the field in tents and those that were convalescent moved into the tent area and the more seriously injured were in the building. We all did double shifts because we had to care for all these patients. And the heat was so unbearable and for the patients in the tents that they -- we did have Italian prisoners of war and they set it up so that they there was -- they put an extra top over the tent and then run cold water over it in order for -- to get it cool. This we -- we stayed in North Africa for one year and we took care of about 5,000 patients during that time.

"Bob Hope came to entertain the troops, came to see troops, 'This Is the Army,' all the shows came. Of course, our social life was wonderful. With a hundred nurses and about a hundred thousand soldiers -- men in the area, we had a wonderful social life. The question was would the Air Force fly us to a dance nearby or the Signal Corps would give us the little meals that they used for their wire for a bedside table for the tents. We had about six nurses that married doctors from the outfit and they set up individual tents for each married couple and that was called Honeymoon Lane. And it was wonderful.

"They got their tents were also with improvised furniture, but most of the fighting was over in Sicily and there was an invasion of Italy. And we followed General Marquardt's Fifth Army and we went up and we were supposed to be sent to Rome, but since the fighting was still going on in Anzio, Rome had not been captured at the time and so we were set up in orange grove outside of Naples near the king's palace.

"And there we took care of originally French colonial troops we had no interpreters or anything, so we were taking care of Arabs and

Senegalese and it was quite an experience taking care of these, their sanitary habits were not the best. And you'd see somebody missing from their bed after surgery and wonder where they were and they're outside using the outside tent as a urinal. So it was quite an experience. But following that, we did get American soldiers wounded from the Anzio beachhead and Casino, the Battle of Casino.

"We stayed in Italy about nine months. We were able to get leave now and then. We went to the Isle of Capri, which was quite an experience. We visited there and various places in Italy and it was very interesting. When we left Italy, then we were transported to France after the invasion of France, and went through the port -- the Southern France through the Port of Marseilles and then on to a Aix-en-Provence. All this time we had been living in tents and when we arrived in Aix-en-Provence, to our great delight, they took over a resort hotel and we lived in this resort hotel and they even checked all the staff so that we had a French chef. It was amazing to know what they could do with dried powdered eggs and different Army food. When we were in Aix-en-Provence, at May 7th, 1945, I believe, that's when VE Day and we were taking part of the VE Day parade. They invited all of the troops, foreign troops, American, British, French troops to march in the VE Day parade. We were in our full uniform marching down the street and all of a sudden I looked up at one of the lampposts and hanging from the lamppost was a man with a big sign across his chest saying 'Collaborator.' They had hung the collaborators. And, of course, it was a horrifying sight to see him swinging from the lamppost. There were several of them.

"At the end of the parade, they had all the women who had consorted with the Germans, head shaved and made them march at the end of the parade to the -- the people watching the parade throwing rocks and stones at them. It was quite an experience to be in that parade. Since there was not very much action after VE Day, we were so short I worked in the orthopedic section taking care of orthopedic patients, but in Italy, they were so short of nurse anesthetists that they decided to train two nurses to become anesthetists, you know, just on-the-job training.

"We had a major who was an anesthesiologist and he took over the job of teaching us anesthesia. So they chose myself and one other, you know, another friend of mine, to become nurse anesthetists. We -- we were doing that for the last year and a half that I was in the Service. I was a nurse administered ether and mostly Pentothal, Sodium Pentothal. And then after that, they -- since, as I said, there were very little action, there were just people evacuated or hurt in automobile accidents, Jeep accidents, something like that.

"So they decided those anesthetists were on the front line, you know, in the evac hospitals and the first aid stations and all those should get a break. So they said -- they -- these people could go to Paris for a training course. They suggested that one nurse anesthetist be sent from each hospital in the area. Well, my friend were -- one friend was getting married, one of the nurse anesthetists, the other friend was having a big romance at the time and so they pleaded with me to go to Paris. And, of course, it was such a hardship for me to go to Paris and spend six weeks there that I reluctantly agreed. They -- I was sent to a station hospital there and the duty was in the morning from 9:00 to 11:00, we either had one lecture for an hour and then we observed the anaesthetist there for the other hour. Then we were free. We had the rest of the day to explore Paris.

"So for six weeks we would leave in the morning about 12:00 noon and then take the subway in Paris and go to the heart of the city. And then just wander. I had a wonderful time just wandering through and not as a tourist, but just to see Paris and you should see it. At the end of this time when I got back to my hospital in Aix-en-Provence, then I became -- we -- we got our orders in August and I think it was August 27th of 1945 to close our hospital. And we transported and sent any patients that we had to other hospitals. In September, we got our orders. We were overseas 28 months and we got our orders to go home. And this was really a wonderful experience.

"So in September, we went -- went on the transport ship the 'General Steward,' and came home. The best sight we ever had was that Statue of Liberty and we were home and were able to go to visit our family once more. And then we got our final -- I think we were discharged from the Army in December of 1945."[103]

World War II was the catalyst for many innovations in the treatment of battlefield trauma wounds. It also led to the transformation of the pharmaceutical industry, the development of the modern air transportation system, the introduction of the helicopter, and major advances in the medical field of psychiatry. This was also the war that saw the advent and use of the most terrifying, devastating weapon ever developed by mankind, the atomic bomb, which was first used against Japan in August 1945.

American Army nurse Ruth Haas had been working with her unit in the Philippines caring for U.S. and Filipino soldiers, and then treating American POWs being liberated from Japanese captivity. At that time they were building up medical teams to cope with the eventual expected invasion of Japan. When World War Two ended with the formal surrender of Japan in September 1945, Ruth was with a group of Army nurses stationed overseas waiting for an assignment. Two months later in November 1945, she was airlifted to Kure, a major naval base there. One day they got an opportunity to relieve the boredom and do a little impromptu sightseeing, but they didn't expect to see the sheer scale of destruction caused by the atomic bomb that fell on Hiroshima. "Get up. We're going on a field trip. Beautiful weather. I remember we walked around. I went into a basement of a house that was no longer there. There wasn't much to see. Buildings in Manila that had been destroyed in the fighting in the Philippines at least left rubble. I didn't see even that in Hiroshima. The nothingness that was there. The realization of what had happened. They had just destroyed everything, it was just the feeling of everything gone. My metal watchband turned black after the trip. We just polished them up because people weren't worried about radiation at that point. You wouldn't want it to happen, to have it dropped but if we would have had to invade Japan, there would've been mass casualties.

---

[103] In Times of War: Memoirs of a World War II Nurse. By Isabelle Cook. (Ivy Pub., 1999).

Anything that ended the war was acceptable. Hopefully, it will never happen again."[104]

World War II casualties both military and civilian were completely unprecedented. No previous war in history had experienced more people killed or more property destroyed. After eight years of war in the Far East, six years of fighting in Europe, the largest war in human history was finally over. Although statistics are often contradictory, and even today it is still difficult to say precisely how many people perished during the war. The final tally in human life is currently estimated at 7.5 million Soviet troops, 3.5 million Germans, 1.25 million Japanese, 452,000 British and Commonwealth, and around 295,000 American service personnel. Exact figures for other allied armies vary. Civilian deaths exceeded military. At least nineteen million Soviet civilians, ten million Chinese, and six million European Jews lost their lives during the war.

The end of World War II would directly and indirectly shape world history for the next five decades. This period is known as the postwar era and was dominated by what became known as the Cold War. It was also dominated with fervent anti-communist sentiment spurred by Senator Joseph McCarthy, which rocked American society to its foundations. One of the major events that occurred as a direct consequence of World War II was the Korean War that emerged from the partition of that country at the end of 1945.

---

[104] "Army Nurse Ruth Hass Saw a Flattened Hiroshima 69 Years Ago," Twin Cities (Pioneer Press, August 13, 2014), https://www.twincities.com/2014/08/13/army-nurse-ruth-hass-saw-a-flattened-hiroshima-69-years-ago/.wel.

CHAPTER SIXTEEN

A Career from Korea

Robert Altman's 1970 movie *M*A*S*H* was set in the Korean War, but it was obvious to all but the poorly informed that it was ostensibly about the Vietnam War. The screenplay was based on the 1968 book *M*A*S*H*, a novel about three Army doctors by Richard Hooker. All of the *M*A*S*H* books written from 1974 through 1997 were co-authored by William E. Butterworth (military novelist W.E.B. Griffin). Richard Hooker was a pseudonym. His real name was H. Richard Hornberger from Bremen, Maine, and he based his fictional books on his real-life experiences as a doctor at the 8055th M.A.S.H. in Korea.

The 8055th was the first medical unit to arrive in Busan, Korea, on July 6, 1950, whereupon it established a sixty-bed hospital. Hornberger claimed that Hawkeye Pierce the show's main character was a loose portrayal of himself. The nurse who inspired the character of "Hotlips Houlihan" was based on Capt. Ruth Dickson, Chief Nurse of the 8055th. But there is another possible contender by the name of "Hotlips Hammerly"—who was by all accounts a bit of an eye pleaser—of the same disposition, and like Dickson she was also from El Paso, Texas. Both were career Army nurses who achieved high ranks.

Hollywood actor Jamie Farr, who played the cross-dressing Corporal Klinger, wasn't the only member of the cast who actually served in Korea, albeit a few years after the war had ended. Alan Alda joined the Army Reserve after graduating from Fordham University in 1956. He then joined the Army reserve and completed a minimum six-month tour of duty as a gunnery officer in Korea. Although some websites erroneously claim he participated in the war, Alda was only fourteen years old when it broke out. Either way, thanks to the Korean War, they all had relatively successful acting careers.

Europe was in no mood to indulge another war it was far too preoccupied with the process of rebuilding and repairing the damage inflicted during World War II. Countries had been devastated, and the dreams, hopes, and aspirations of millions had been destroyed or simply eradicated. America had the bomb and had more than aptly demonstrated they were not afraid to use it. Meanwhile, affluent 1950s America witnessed a dramatic surge of anti-communist sentiment fueled by the likes of one particular minor, self-aggrandizing republican named Joseph McCarthy. He was a man with a mission, a drinking problem, and a chip on his shoulder as big as Mount Rushmore. For the entertainment industry it was a time of terror and betrayal at the hands of America's latter day version of the Spanish Inquisition, the House Un-American Activities Committee (HUAC).

But this minor politician overextended his pernicious tentacles in 1953 when McCarthy accused the U.S. military of harboring communists in 1953, it led to his downfall. CBS TV commentator Edward R. Murrow publicly denounced McCarthy's errant tactics and condemned HUAC as a threat to American's core democratic values. In December 1954, one year after the Korean War ended, the Senate officially reproached McCarthy for "conduct unbecoming a senator." They were dangerous and volatile times indeed.

During the first months of his presidency, Harry Truman's administration dispatched General Douglas MacArthur to command the United Nations forces. The Korean conflict lasted three long years (1950–1953).

It was punctuated by self-serving negotiations and stalemates that only served to stall the armistice and devour thousands of lives.

Native American Marjorie Montgomery Lovelady was a nurse attached to a M.A.S.H. unit during the Korean War. "I went in the operating room at 0530 one morning and didn't leave for 72 hours. We treated at least 2,000 wounded, everything from minor to major injuries. Minor injuries were when fingers or parts of hands were blown off. Major injuries were soldiers with "half their head blown away, legs blown off, terrible burns, chests blown open. For three days and three nights we didn't leave the operating room. When the temperature dropped to -20c they gave us whiskey to keep the blood circulating in our legs and feet and they yelled "stomp those feet ". While working with M.A.S.H. units at Pusan, Seoul, Chosin Reservoir and other sites she came to be known by her Cherokee name 'Many Tears'. She said, "After boot camp, I thought that I wanted to sign up for 20 years, after four years, that was enough. I'd seen enough blood and guts. Many call it a police action. But it had bombs, bullets, tents, and chaos. It was a bloody war. I was a complete basket case after the war. I was very traumatized, a misfit in society. I still have flashbacks, but I can handle it. "I don't take medicine for trauma but try to work it out. Every time I said Korea, people would spit on me, call me name. They said I should have died with the rest. It was never recognized as a war. That's just a disgrace. I saw lots of young soldiers die, but you know who had the worst jobs? The officers. They examined the wounded and said, 'Put them at the end of the line.' They knew we were running short on blood. They said to give them morphine and let them ease on out. They were not in pain. We gave them morphine for suffering. Made me so mature. I have so much pride and dignity in the honor of serving my country. Even though I was just a nurse and played a small part I'm glad I'm a vet and served in Korea. And if I could do it over again, I'd do it just like I did then."

The Korean War is often referred to as America's "forgotten war." It was in essence a component part of a larger Cold War struggle to extinguish the same communism that McCarthy had so fervently attempted to expose and destroy. For those who found themselves embroiled in this bitter conflict it will never be forgotten. The combat that occurred in the Korean peninsula was in many ways comparable to anything that happened in WWII. There are still omnipresent tensions between the north and south, and there is still a very clear danger that these could easily transpose to all-out war at any moment. The disparity between the two halves of this troubled peninsula is simply too great. The south is an economic powerhouse, a super state that has championed technical innovation to become one of the world's leading manufacturers of consumer durables. Meanwhile the north remains subjugated by a volatile, repressive regime, which has no place in this day and age.

Communist North Korean forces invaded South Korea on June 27, 1950. The United Nations Security Council retaliated by approving a resolution proposed by the United States calling for armed force to repel the North Korean invaders. The action provided the pretext for U.S. intervention in the conflict and was the first time in its young history that the Security Council had approved the use of military force. The U.N. called on member nations to "render such assistance to the Republic of Korea as may be necessary to repel the armed attack and to restore international peace and security to the area."[105] Before any action was taken on the part of the U.N. in regards to authorizing intervention in the Korean War, the U.S. had already dispatched military support to prop up the weak South Korean army on June 27, 1950. The war would develop into a fearsome protracted slogging match that culminated in bitter stalemate, and a war without a viable peace.

By this time major advances in military medicine and battlefield healthcare had been developed. Now the allies would be able to call on the services of the Mobile Army Surgical Hospital (M.A.S.H.) units. The purpose of these units was to provide the wounded with surgical care in as close proximity as was reasonably possible to the battlefront. Battlefield experiences in WWII proved that wounded personnel suffered if there was a delay in providing definitive treatment of their injuries. The establishment of the Mobile Army Surgical Hospital was announced on

---

[105] Encyclopedia of the United Nations and International Agreements: G to M. By Edmund Jan Osmańczyk.

August 23, 1945, at the very end of WWII. This would be the first war where helicopters were regularly used as flying ambulances to transport the injured to better provisioned medical facilities in the shortest time possible. Innovative new techniques such as plastic utility bags and the national blood banking program saved countless lives. Effective body armor was developed to allow better mobility while offering protection. These radical improvements not only saved the lives of soldiers in combat, they were soon adopted by the civilian sector.

Dr. Elliott Cutler, Brigadier General and consultant to the Surgeon General, said, "I would even urge an extension of this forward surgery, believing surgery should be brought to the soldier, not the soldier to the surgeon."[106] It looked good on paper, but when the Korean War broke out these units were woefully unprepared. There were only 156 Medical Corps officers in the U.S. 8th Army but 346 was the authorized strength. It was immediately necessary to staff the 8054th evacuation hospital and the 8055th, 8063rd, and 8076th M.A.S.H.s. Reserves were mobilized and in June of 1950, owing to a shortage of doctors in the U.S. Army Medical Corps, the government instituted a "doctor draft." At that time very few U.S. military medical units had any experience in northeast Asia. Colonel Chauncey Dovell, 8th U.S. Army surgeon, quickly dispatched M.A.S.H. units to Korea to provide medical support. Consequently, eight M.A.S.H. units were able to deploy rapidly, and it didn't take them long to adapt to the rugged terrain on the peninsula. One of the doctors to get called up during the doctor draft was Robert L. Emanuele. He started out at Camp Atterbury that had been the staging post for many U.S. divisions in WWII. As a result of the doctor draft, he was among the chosen.

"The thought of going to Korea scared me to death. It wasn't so much that I feared getting injured or even killed, but what really worried me was that I might not be a good enough doctor to provide the lifesaving skills that our soldiers would need. After a few weeks of training at Camp Atterbury in Indiana, I was sent to Korea, assigned as a surgeon with the 8209th MASH (Mobile Army Surgical Hospital) Unit. I arrived at the

---

[106] Activities of Surgical Consultants, Volume 2. By United States. Army Medical Service (United States. Army Medical Dept.).

unit the morning of Sept. 22, 1951. MASH units were designed to be mobile and operate close to the battlefield, and the 8209th was about 10 miles from the front when I arrived. I remember hearing the sounds of artillery shells in the distance and thinking 'Wow, this really is happening.' I don't recall much of that first day, but I do remember being cold and homesick my first night. One of the nurses brought me a sweater and blanket. The blanket was from Marshall Field & Co. Strange what you remember.

"Almost every day there was work to do. It would always start with the announcement over the camp's public address system of 'incoming wounded.' This was quickly followed by the sound of 'choppers' coming in. I recall our unit had four helicopters. There were many examples of heroic acts in Korea, but the helicopter pilots were heroic on every flight. They would pluck wounded soldiers from the battlefield, sometimes under heavy fire. I was always amazed how brave those pilots were.

"The workdays were long, 12 hours on and 12 hours off, and the work was a constant challenge in terms of the sheer volume of cases and in the complexity and variety of wounds. Out of necessity, we often operated solo, with the assistance of a nurse or medical technician.

"The wounds could be horrific. A common injury was the result of an anti-personnel mine known as the 'Bouncing Betty.' When tripped, it fired straight up about three feet before it exploded, usually disemboweling or maiming those unfortunate enough to be within range. It was a horrible weapon. A lot of the surgery we did was on the lower extremity, doing our best to repair eviscerated abdomens and slaughtered lower limbs.

"The work was also emotionally challenging. I remember one particular case where a young soldier had been badly injured. Myself, Ray (Capt. Ray Crissy) and Mert (Maj. Merton White) worked on him for hours. We had opened his chest when his heart just stopped beating. We did everything we could to keep him alive, including injecting blood directly into his aorta and massaging his heart. I still remember the feeling of holding his heart in my hand. We were able to bring him back and I remember joking with him a few days later. He seemed to be doing well and I really thought he was going to make it. But his kidneys ultimately failed and we lost him. Like so many of the GIs, he was nice kid whose life ended way too early.

"Korea was not all work and we definitely had fun too, although not quite to the extent portrayed on the 'M*A*S*H' television series. Our living quarters were tight with six men to a tent. I was lucky and got along really well with the other five guys. Three of us were from the Chicago area, and to make it seem a little more like home we painted signs on the door and inside the tent naming it the 'Drake Hotel.' We had fun with that and would often answer the phone 'Drake Hotel.' We had a potbelly stove to keep the place warm and would try to cook all sorts of things—from pizza to apple pie. On a few occasions I can remember us 'hotel dwellers' preparing dinner for the nurses. We would make a big deal out of that. We would serve drinks, dinner and play music on an old phonograph. Maybe dance a little too. It was a lot of fun, but also a way for us to say 'thank you' for the work they did—which went way beyond nursing. They would assist in surgery, suture wounds and start transfusions. They really were true medical professionals."[107]

The M*A*S*H TV series didn't endear everyone. Some Korean War veterans objected vociferously to its humorous content, but that didn't stop the show from becoming hugely successful. Twenty years after the Korean War ended, physician Dale Drake and his wife, Cathy (who both served at the 8055th M.A.S.H.), helped Hollywood transform the way America envisaged the Korean War by relating some personal experiences and portraying the lives of the medical staff, military personnel, and patients who passed through a fictional M.A.S.H unit. Cathy (neé McDonough) Drake first arrived in Korea in 1950 as part of the Army Nurse Corp at the 8076th M.A.S.H. before the unit was dispatched to Pyongyang in North Korea. When the Chinese hordes crossed the border, she returned to Japan and was later assigned back to South Korea.

---

107 Robert L Emanuele, "Memories of 'M*A*S*H' by a Real-Life MASH Doctor - Near West," Chicago Tribune, https://digitaledition.chicagotribune.com/tribune/article_popover.aspx?guid=71b8382d-45da-4995-845a-1c9f3975dbdf.

That's when she went to work for the 8055th M.A.S.H. unit, right on the 38th parallel and the place where she met her future husband, Dale.

"'I was an army nurse stationed in Walter Reed Hospital in Washington, D.C., and I got assigned to the 171st Evacuation Hospital in Korea,' Cathy said. 'I went from Fort Bragg to California, and then we sailed to Tokyo. The 171st Evac was a big hospital, and I was sent over to one of the five MASH units they had in Korea. That's where one of the doctors, an anesthesiologist, was waiting for his replacement to come, and he told me 'Now that would be a nice guy for you, Cathy.'"[108]

The anesthesiologist was referring to Dale Drake, who was the replacement. While Dale was working as a chief anesthesiologist in Arkansas, he had joined the Army Reserve and in 1951 he was issued with orders to join the Far East Command, whereupon he was assigned to the 8055th.

The Korean War was a tragic fratricidal conflict that inflicted corrosive and lasting wounds on the peninsula and can be correctly regarded in retrospect as one of the most destructive wars of the 20th century. It is estimated that as many as three million Koreans died, at least half of them were civilians. It was the war that established the American base structure abroad and a national security state at home, because defense[109] spending nearly quadrupled in the last six months of 1950. While South Korea adopted democracy and capitalism, North Korea remains today one of the most stringent and isolated communist states in the world. The Korean War is most definitely not forgotten.

---

[108] Louis La Plante, "More M*A*S*H," Evansville Living Magazine (July/August 2010), http://www.evansvilleliving.com/articles/more-mash.

[109] https://www.jcs.mil/Portals/36/Documents/History/Policy/Policy_V003_P001.pdf.

CHAPTER SEVENTEEN

Medevac in Vietnam

While the 1950s was a time of great prosperity and everything was in abundance in the United States, the 1960s witnessed a time of seismic social and cultural upheaval. Young Americans had witnessed the assassination of a president, the rise of the black civil rights movement, hippies and their psychedelic lifestyles, and music from the British "invasion." It was a time of unprecedented change. African American college students staged sit-ins, freedom rides, and protest marches to challenge segregation south of the Mason Dixon line. Their efforts led the federal government to pass the Civil Rights Act of 1964, prohibiting discrimination in public facilities and employment, and the 24th Amendment and the Voting Rights Act of 1965, guaranteeing voting rights.

Youth culture was empowered and enhanced by the copious availability of marijuana, LSD, and free love, even if the latter was just an excuse for ugly men to "make love not war" to beautiful women. In retrospect hippies could have been an abbreviation of hypocrites because these ersatz libertines didn't share much love with returning Vietnam veterans. During WWII an infantryman could expect to have spent at least ten days in combat in the course of one year. In Vietnam that could have been up to 240 days in almost constant combat in the course of one year. In August 1964, in response to an alleged attack by North Vietnamese patrol boats on U.S. destroyers in the Gulf of Tonkin Congress passed the "Gulf of Tonkin Resolution," which unanimously authorized President Lyndon Johnson to wage an undeclared war in Vietnam.

The war was referred to as a police action just as the Korean War had been. The word "alleged" is significant here. When Commander Stockdale in charge of the ship Ticonderoga later reported, "I had the best seat in the house to watch that event and our destroyers were just shooting at phantom targets, there were no PT boats there, there was nothing there but black water and American firepower." Another captain deduced that these so-called attacks were actually the results of "overeager sonar operators" and questionable equipment performance. No torpedoes had actually been detected throughout the whole encounter. U.S. Navy operators were probably hearing the ships propellers reflecting off her rudder during sharp turns. This was the premise that provided Johnson with the authority to send United States troops to Vietnam.

Vietnam delineated a whole generation. To the uninformed it was rock and roll meets napalm, and to those who survived it Vietnam left an enduring, often tragic legacy. The main protagonists were the "baby boomers" whose fathers fought World War II for a better world. They were raised on a tangible diet of fervent patriotism, anti-communism, Audie Murphy, John Wayne, and a veritable host of indomitable heroes to emulate and admire.

Vietnam veteran Jim Truesdale said that he was in DaNang when the north launched the Tet offensive in 1968, "As soon as someone shouted 'Incoming', total chaos erupted, mortar bombs and NVA shells were landing everywhere inside our perimeter blowing everything to hell. My C.O. began handing out flak jackets to the troops for protection. The problem was, these flak jackets had been specially made for the South Vietnamese Army, and consequently our guys couldn't get them on. They were completely useless to us. That kind of sums up the American experience of Vietnam. We had the equipment, we had the men and they were the best but with no cohesive plan and subject to constant political intervention there was no way that we could have ever have come out on top."

Then the west had the media to contend with. Some of the most prolific and unambiguous images beamed around the world were of civilian casualties being airlifted in Bell "Huey" helicopters, accompanied by whirring rotor blades and small arms popping in all directions. For the young Americans who were drafted, it wasn't about the political machinations of corrupt governments or polarized ideologies. Their service hinged on one pervasive question: "Am I going to make it out of here?" Whether they would or not would depended on two primal factors: the severity of the wound and the effectiveness of the medical treatment they received when that wound was inflicted.

Ron 'Bev' Donahey was a medic attached to Alpha Company 2/8th Infantry. He was there in the heat of the fighting; his recollections vividly describe the experience of what it was really like to be a combat medic in Vietnam. His testimony proves irrefutably that the courageous American's who served there were the same caliber as those who had fought in previous wars, he recounted, "The jungle was so thick that the choppers were having difficulty getting the dead and wounded out. Our fire support base had been firing continuously since around midnight. Over fifteen hundred rounds had been fired in support of Bravo and Charlie-Companies. There was also a group from the 25th Infantry Division being hit as well. They were about two klicks east of the firebase, and had picked up a lot of injured, and had some KIA's. One medevac chopper was shot down, killing all seven on board.

"As soon as the sun was up, the Air Force came in full strength. A-1E Skyraiders and Phantom jets were everywhere dropping napalm and five hundred-pound bombs. Huey gunships could be seen circling at a distance, waiting for their turn. Occasionally, a Huey would land inside our perimeter to inspect bullet holes they had received.

"Word came down that reinforcements were desperately needed for Bravo Company. They were surrounded and could not move until the NVA broke contact. It was decided that Alpha Company would send its 3rd platoon and one squad from weapons platoon. We were to leave as soon as possible. Third platoon's medic was in base camp, so I began to prepare to take his place. I loaded my rucksack with extra medical supplies and waited along with the others until around 1500 that afternoon. We boarded Hueys and took off. Because of snipers, we had to circle for twenty minutes until it was safe enough to go in. The hill was just large enough for one chopper to come down at a time.

"When I landed, I saw my good friend Harold Stenseth crouching in a foxhole. He looked very tired and was just as glad to see me as I was to see him. When I got to his foxhole I began to smell an odor I had never smelled before. A sweet pungent odor that made me nauseated at first. Lying all around the perimeter were NVA bodies already decaying in the heat and humidity of the afternoon.

"I couldn't spend much time talking because we only had a couple of hours to prepare our own positions for the night. I began digging with the Lieutenant and Sgt. Moran. We were able to dig a position large enough for all three of us to kneel comfortably and have our bodies below ground. We had brought in lots of sand bags, which we used to fortify our hole. I positioned some sandbags and put my aid bag behind them, so I could grab it when I had to go.

"As darkness came, everyone seemed prepared. Our position was half way down the hill, and just behind us were my guys from weapons platoon. Fifty feet below us was the perimeter, the first line of defense, and directly in front of us was a machine gun position. The rest of Alpha Company was inserted into the perimeter. The hill was sloped just enough that we could fire over the others without fear of hitting one of our own.

"We had decided on a casualty collection point on top of the hill, and although we were still a medic short, we felt we were ready. Harold's position was a hundred feet away and to my left. Throughout the day, we had placed squad size observation posts out in front of us on all sides. Now that darkness had come, the world was ghostly silent around us. The three-man listening post slipped silently out of the perimeter and were soon lost in the blackness. The LP's were to be an advanced warning system in case the enemy began sneaking up on us. The LP's would go out with a radio, their weapons, and a claymore mine or two, and stay there until morning, or until the enemy got too close. If they had to come in during the night they were to explode their claymores, and make sure they brought the radio and their weapons.

"The NVA usually did not attack early in the evening, so we were pretty sure it would not happen for a few hours. We went on half alert until midnight, and then full alert from then on. The CP was close to our position, and occasionally, we could hear the radio. The fire support base knew exactly where we were, and every so often the Artillery Forward Observer (FO) would have them fire some rounds around us just in case the enemy was close. It wasn't a matter of hiding from anyone. Charley knew exactly where we were, so it was just a matter of waiting until we got hit.

"In the distance, we could hear the muffled sounds of artillery being fired in support of Charlie Company. A full moon was shining under scattered clouds, and our eyes had adjusted to the darkness of the night. It was now over four hours since the sun had gone down, and I doubt if anyone was sleeping. It was very peaceful.

"Our listening posts began to report sounds of movement. The brief transmissions had been tinged with panic, a few words, almost frantic description of NVA movement too close for comfort. Suddenly the world of silver moonbeams and soft grays was transformed into one of moving shadows. The tranquil beauty of the night was shattered as the North Vietnamese began their attack. Their tracers etched brilliant green streaks through the blackness, as they seemed to float towards us like glowing baseballs. The calm of the jungle was now broken by the concussions of our own artillery and claymore mines. The rattle of machine guns, and M-16's was punctuated by the explosions of grenades. Shrapnel and bullets slammed into the jungle like the rains of the monsoons. Mixed with this confusion was the sound of AK-47's. A sound I was to become familiar with before my tour was completed.

"Shadows cast from trip flares silhouetted enemy soldiers as they moved just inside the tree line. The moment I had thought about for eleven months had arrived. My first experience with combat had begun, and with it came an urgent call from just in front of us for a medic.

"As I jumped out of the hole, Lt. Underwood grabbed my arm and said, 'Doc, take my .45.' I told him I never needed it and took off. As I slid and crawled down to the perimeter, I could see twinkling lights, like fireflies, pointed at us only a hundred feet away. Occasionally an explosion from a Chicom grenade would cause me to duck. Our machine gun was laying down a steady stream of red tracers. At least it wasn't that position that needed help.

"As I neared the perimeter, the firing in front of me began to slow and finally came to a stop. Not one bullet was coming in or going out, yet the rest of the perimeter was a continual sound of battle. The fire support base had their rhythm going and was putting a steady flow of artillery around us.

"I came to a position and asked who called for a medic. When I realized it was the machine gun position, I thought, 'Good choice, Donahey. The one gun the enemy wanted most, and you had to stop here.' At that moment, the moon came out from behind a cloud, to reveal in sharp relief a body lying face down out in the field of fire just feet from the tree line.

"Without thinking, I ran out to it. When I got to him he whispered to me to stay down. The person who had shot him was in the trees just about 10 feet or so away. I asked him where he was hit, and he said it felt like his hip. I could see a blood stain, so I gave him a shot of morphine and crawled back to the machine gun position. I told the guys I needed help, and one of the guys jumped up and we ran back out. We each grabbed a shoulder and a leg and ran back inside our perimeter.

"When we reached the top of the hill, the perimeter where we had just been erupted into fighting once again. As we reached the collection point, Harold came towards me carrying someone else wrapped in a poncho. I asked him if it was one of his guys or one of mine, and he said he thought it was one of mine. I knelt beside the body and recognized my good friend Larry Harshman. He had been hit in the back of the head with shrapnel from a grenade and was in shock. Even in the moonlight, he looked worse than the training films at Ft. Sam.

"After getting the two wounded bandaged and as comfortable as possible, I headed back to my position. The firing seemed to be tapering off some. When I reached my hole, I asked the Lieutenant if there had been any more calls for a medic. I was glad to learn that there hadn't been. I continued to the perimeter and crawled into a foxhole with two guys from 3rd platoon. It was then I learned that the guy had been in front of us on a three-man listening post, and that only two of the three had made it back inside the perimeter. The other one was still somewhere outside. I asked if anyone knew who it was, and it was believed to be someone from Bravo Company named Kendel Washington.

"The firing had all but stopped by this time. I looked at my watch and realized the battle had raged for almost an hour and it had seemed only a few minutes. It appeared we only had the two WIA's and the MIA. Throughout the night, we could detect movement and noises coming from just inside the tree line. We prayed it was not the enemy grouping for another assault. At this point, all our claymores had been exploded and the trip flares had been used. As the night wore on and we were not attacked again, we realized it was the NVA taking care of their dead and wounded. The artillery continued to plaster the surrounding jungle in an attempt to kill as many as possible.

"I lay in the foxhole thinking of Kendel. At times, I had grandiose thoughts of someone going with me and we could go out and find him. We listened for any sound that might have been him but heard nothing.

"As the skies began to get light, a squad formed and headed towards the listening post. They found Kendel still leaning against the same tree he had been at when the attack began. His hands were raised in a grotesque attempt to ward off the danger. He was riddled from his neck to his abdomen with machine gun bullets. At least he had died instantly.

"The squad also noticed something else. The listening post had made a deadly error. They had returned to the same spot as the observation post had been. During the time between the two, the enemy had taken vines from the trees, and tied them to use as hand railings. They quietly crept up to the end of the vines and knew they were just ten feet in front of the listening post. All they had to do was open fire. We were fortunate to get the other two guys back at all.

"I returned to the top of the hill to see if Larry had lived through the night. It had been a rough night for him. There had been moments when he would come to and try to get up and run but would slip once more into the coma. We had called for a chopper to come at first light, and in the distance, I could hear the muffled sounds of the medevac as it slipped through the moisture laden air. As long as the cloud ceiling remained where it was, and we could keep the snipers away, the chopper could land, giving Larry and the other guy the chance to live.

"I looked towards the sound and saw three choppers coming in fast. As they neared, two split off and I could see they were gunships sent along for protection. The medevac approached the landing area in a steep, fast decent. I saw one of the door gunners, standing on the strut, firing at the ridge they had just crossed. Then they were on the ground.

"As soon as they touched down we were running forward with our two WIA's and the one KIA. All the while the door gunners hovered over their M-60 machine guns, and the gunships circled overhead, as we loaded the wounded on the Huey. The rotors began to turn faster and faster as the pilot prepared for lift-off. I touched Larry's hand, and looked into his eyes, but there was nothing. He had slipped into a coma once more. The chopper lifted to a hover, and once the pilot felt sure the load was not too heavy he increased the pitch of the main rotor and was on his way to the 18th Surgical Hospital in Pleiku.

"I stood there and watched the chopper as it became a dot on the horizon and was soon out of sight. I turned and looked out over the field of fire in front of our perimeter and saw the new bodies that had not been there when darkness had come the night before.

"As I stood there, my friends from weapons platoon came up to me and one of them asked if I was all right. Then another one said they couldn't believe what I had done the night before. They had watched as I had gone outside the perimeter to get the wounded guy, and had known both of us were going to be killed before we could get back in. They had then realized the enemy was not firing on that section of the perimeter at all. My friend Bob Stockton said that if I was ever in Chicago he was going to buy me the biggest steak that city had. As we stood there looking at each other, the Lieutenant walked up and told me he was glad nothing had happened. He too had watched and expected the enemy to open up and kill us both. He then said he was going to put me in for a Bronze Star.

"I went looking for Harold and found him sitting by his foxhole looking like I felt. I never said anything, just sat down beside him. What had seemed like hours last night had lasted only a little over fifty minutes. It is not easy to gauge time accurately when death is walking beside you. We sat there gazing out in front of us, watching the guys inspecting the bodies, and finally decided to look, too.

"I walked out into the killing zone in front of our positions, and there, among a dozen or more bodies covered with giant black flies, and maggots already eating away at the flesh, I realized I was witnessing a real war. Not something far away or something I was not involved with. What I was involved with was the senseless destruction of human lives.

"I knelt beside one of the bodies, which only hours before had been a young North Vietnamese. I looked at his face and saw the horror of violence, not the peace he should have had. I opened his pack and saw the plastic shaving gear. The kind you would buy your son at the Five and Dime store. A letter half finished, and pictures of a young mother holding a child. He had a spoon and fork he had made from a piece of aluminum.

"I was looking through a dead man's earthly possessions. A dead man whose family would never know what happened to him. They would only know that he never returned from the war. I moved from one body to the next. The type of wounds varied. Some were missing limbs and others where hardly recognizable as once being healthy young men.

"We were tired, and both felt we would rather be somewhere else. Nothing much had changed since yesterday. We were still surrounded on a hill few people knew about, and fewer still would ever hear about. A hill that meant nothing to anyone. A hill we would hopefully walk away from soon, never to return.

"Throughout the day, we tried to cover the bloating bodies of the dead NVA as best we could. We knew we weren't going to get rid of the smell, but we were willing to try anything. All the time we had to be careful because of snipers. Choppers came on a regular basis all day long and by evening we had all the supplies we needed. Empty ammo boxes were everywhere.

"The medic from Bravo Company that had been in base camp showed up on one of the choppers, so we were finally up to full strength. I moved in with Harold, and we tried to enlarge his foxhole to fit both of us. It was mostly rock, so we weren't very successful. He is a couple of inches shorter than I am so when we both got in the foxhole we had to lay on our sides and I would have to bend my knees a little. We positioned logs and sandbags over the top of us, leaving a small opening to get out. This gave us added protection from grenades and shrapnel. The enemy must have run out of mortars because we had not had any more hit our perimeter since the first night.

"During the late afternoon, Harold and I had a chance to relax. As we sat on the edge of our position talking, I noticed for the first time just how close the bodies were. Harold said the NVA must have been very close to them as they tried to get to high ground the first day. No sooner had they arrived on the hill and positioned the observation posts, they were hit.

"The OP directly in front of where he had begun to dig his foxhole was immediately overrun. He looked up and saw two of the three guys from the OP trying to make it to the perimeter. One of the two was trying to drag the other. It looked like the guy's leg had more than one knee joint. The third guy was also wounded and was being held captive by the NVA just inside the tree line. The enemy had positioned themselves around him and every so often would poke him with a stick or their AK-47's. When he began calling for help, Harold and two others started out of the perimeter to get him. Suddenly Harold found himself lying flat on his back. His first thought was he had been hit. He looked up and he saw 46 year old platoon sergeant Charles Turner he realized he had been tackled. Sgt. Turner told them to stay where they were and taking off his shirt he began to fill it with grenades and M-16 ammo. Lt. Hunter saw what was happening and took his shirt off and began doing the same thing.

"The NVA had positioned a machine gun just inside the trees about fifty feet away from where Harold was laying. They had expected someone to come directly out of the perimeter and try to rescue him. Instead Sgt. Turner and Lt. Hunter did an end run and came in behind them, catching the NVA completely by surprise.

"With Sgt. Turner leading the way, they attacked with grenades, grabbed the wounded guy, and made it into the perimeter without being injured. On the way in they had knocked out the machine gun position, which was just in front of Harold.

"Harold had been trying to work on the guy with the wounded leg and now that the machine gun was out of commission he was able to examine the wounds a little closer. There were numerous bullet wounds plus all three major bones in his left leg appeared to be shattered. He was losing a lot of blood and it was important to get the bleeding stopped.

"After giving a shot of morphine, Harold positioned the guy half over himself and was using his own legs as a brace. He was doing this while lying on his back. Whenever he would try to rise, another enemy machine gun would fire a burst over them.

"Directly in front of Harold, and maybe seventy-five feet away, lay the machine gun that Sgt. Turner had knocked out. In a desperate attempt to retrieve the gun, the NVA sent one after another out to get it. In the end, seventeen had tried, and all seventeen had died.

"They were the pile of bodies that now lay just in front of our position. It appeared they had been stacked there but they had just fallen over one another as they died. We looked at them and wondered how many more would die before we were able to get off the hill.

"Small patrols had gone out during the day to see what was in the jungle around us. They could only get a couple of hundred meters out before they would begin to receive sniper fire, so we knew we were still surrounded. On their way back into the perimeter, one of the patrols captured an NVA sergeant. During the interrogation, he claimed he had gotten separated from his patrol and said that the NVA were going to try to overrun us. More soldiers were on their way from a camp just across the Cambodian border. He said a lot of his men had been killed and they wanted to pay us back.

"These patrols had found bodies tied to bamboo poles, which allowed the enemy to carry their dead away. A lot of broken weapons littered the jungle surrounding our perimeter, and blood trails indicated the enemy had taken a terrible loss.

"We had been very fortunate the night before and we knew it. We were filled with apprehension as we thought about what the enemy prisoner had told us and of the darkness which was just a couple of hours away. When sunset came, we were as ready as we could possibly be.

"Puff the Magic Dragon or Spooky was the names we called the AC-47 gunships. They had been modified by mounting three 7.62 mm General Electric miniguns to fire through two rear window openings and the side cargo door, all on the left side of the aircraft, to provide close air support for ground troops. The aircraft also carried flares it could drop to illuminate the battleground.

"At 2000, Puff showed up to keep us company. He could stay around for a couple of hours at a time, but he assured us that when he had to leave another Puff would be there to take his place.

"At 2030, the listening post directly in front of us began reporting sounds of movement. Their whispered voices indicated that they were extremely frightened and rightfully so. Without warning, all three of them came running into the perimeter. They were very fortunate that our own guns had not killed them as they ran in.

"The procedure for the listening post was simple. They were to stay out until given permission to return or were hit by the enemy. When they did leave their post, they were to blow the claymores and bring the radio and their weapons with them. We now had a slight problem in that two of the three had left their weapons at the listening post and the radio and claymores were still there as well. All three of them were now sitting beside our foxhole and were as frightened as anyone could get.

"Sgt. Turner who had fought in WWII, Korea, and now here in Vietnam came over and sat down beside them and asked what had happened. After listening to their explanation, he reminded them that they would have to go back to their position and get the things they had left behind. The radio especially could not fall into the enemy's hands. If that happened, they could then listen to all our radio communication. He stood up grabbed his M-16 and said he was going with them. It was evident that no one wanted to go but they did not have much choice. What Sgt. Turner had said made sense.

"As they snuck out of the perimeter once again, I wondered if they would live to see the sunrise in the morning. Within a few minutes the radio came to life and we heard Sgt. Turner's voice. They had found the listening post and were going to stay there for a while longer.

"A few minutes later, we heard a voice ask what time it was. Someone said, 'Why, who wants to know' and the voice responded, 'Never mind GI, what time is it?' The problem with this exchange was the voice was coming from somewhere in front of our perimeter. Just then an NVA soldier jumped up and opened fire. He had crawled to within thirty feet of a machine gun position without being detected. He was able to get a couple of rounds off before the machine gun killed him. This was un-nerving to say the least. The clouds had disappeared, and we had a full moon shining and we still had not seen any movement. At this point, we pulled our listening posts in and prepared to fight.

"Puff reported seeing lights coming towards us from three directions. He asked if we could illuminate the perimeter in some way, and he would begin firing his miniguns. With all the empty ammo boxes, it wasn't hard to get some fires going. We had just gotten them started when he told us to get down, the enemy was almost on top of us. He no sooner got the words out of his mouth when all hell broke loose.

"Harold and I lay in our hole watching Puff circle our perimeter five hundred feet above us. The miniguns buzzed like angry bees as lines of red came from them, the shells landing just inside the tree line. Every fifth bullet was a tracer and a gun that can fire fifty-five hundred shells a minute can put on quite a show. The parachute flares cast an eerie glow over us.

"All our claymores and trip flares were used up in the first minutes of the battle. Our perimeter put out a steady flow of fire for the next fifteen minutes. Every once in a while, Puff would get out of the way and the fire support base would saturate the jungle around us with 105mm and 155mm artillery shells.

"We laid in our foxhole waiting for a call for a medic, but none came. In the beginning the tree line had sparkled with the muzzle bursts of AK-47's, grenades, and B-40 rockets. As we lay in our hole, we could hear bullets hitting the logs and sandbags that lay over us, and we could clearly hear shrapnel from our artillery as it sliced across the hill.

"When the firing ended, Harold and I made a quick check of the perimeter and found that no one had been injured. Even with Puff there to help us, it had been an intense battle. It was hard to believe that no one had been hit.

"When we returned from checking each position, I grabbed my poncho liner and stood up to shake it out. Just then an artillery round landed close to the perimeter. When I heard it coming in loud and fast, I dropped to the ground. When I fell, I landed on a small stump, hitting me in the middle of my chest and knocking the wind out of me. Harold was sure I had been hit with shrapnel, so he jumped out of the hole and asked me where I had been hit. Because I couldn't breathe yet I couldn't tell him I had not been hit. He rolled me over and began checking for a wound. At this point I wanted to laugh and cry at the same time. When I was able to tell him what happened, we laid there on the ground and laughed till tears ran down our face.

"Next to us was a three-man position. It was made so they could kneel with their arms resting on the firing ports. At 0300 the guy in the middle left to get more grenades. While he was gone an artillery round exploded somewhere out in front of us and we could hear something swishing through the air towards us. It entered the foxhole and imbedded in the wall right where he would have been kneeling. It was a six-inch, white-hot, jagged piece of shrapnel from the 105mm round. If he had been there, I'm sure it would have killed him.

"As morning came we began to stretch our stiff bodies. A lot of us were extremely tired by this time. Three days without much sleep was beginning to take its toll. The Captain put us on half alert and the rest tried to get some sleep before it got too hot.

"We were sitting by our foxhole talking and watching the choppers come and go when I noticed what looked like a man hiding in a tall tree across the valley half a mile away. Whenever a chopper would come, he would go to the back side of the tree then reappear when it took off. I asked the artillery Lieutenant if I could use his binoculars, and sure enough there was a man in the tree. I handed the binoculars back to the Lieutenant and suggested he look. After seeing the enemy, he got on the radio and called the fire support base.

"The artillery was just getting ready to fire when we saw a Phantom jet fly by with one bomb hanging under a wing. The Lieutenant asked the artillery to hold for a minute while he turned to a different frequency and was soon talking with the pilot. Yes, it was an extra bomb and yes, he would be more than willing to circle back and drop it on a tree.

"As he circled off in the distance, the artillery put a spotter round where we wanted the bomb dropped and then the Phantom began to dive. What a sight to see this jet come falling from the sky then level off and put his five hundred pounder at the base of the tree. When the dust settled, the tree was gone.

"A patrol headed across the valley to check things out. When they returned, we found that the NVA had been digging new mortar pits. The bomb had destroyed the position and the ammo as well. No bodies were found but that was not unusual.

"Around noon a chopper landed and out stepped a news team from NBC. As that chopper took off, another landed and out stepped five high-ranking officers. As the news team began taking their pictures and getting their interviews, the officers began mingling with us. They seemed to be taking our emotional and psychological temperature. One of these officers sat down beside Harold and asked if there was anything he could do for him. Without hesitating Harold told him he could get us off the hill.

"Since the first day on the hill, Bravo Company's CO Captain Alfred Jones had begun calling Sgt. Turner, 'Poppa T' and with great respect for the man, the name had stuck. The Captain told the reporter how 'Poppa T' and Lt. Hunter had saved the guy the first night, and how he had gone out to the listening post the second night. The cameraman took pictures of the battlefield and of us guys who had put up such a successful fight, then they climbed on their chopper and left.

"We had gone all day without a shot being fired at us and as darkness came we hoped we had seen the last of the enemy. Throughout the night, we could only hear the normal jungle noises and the listening posts reported no movement at all. Puff returned around 2100 but things were so quiet he finally left and went back to Pleiku.

"When the sun came up, we were told to prepare to leave. We were going to try walking off the hill. The perimeter was not large enough for an LZ, so we had no choice but to walk away. This brought mixed emotions because the perimeter had been rather safe after the first night. It afforded us a feeling of security, which we were not willing to give up easily. As soon as we left its safety, we would become vulnerable once again.

"We sent a squad size point out ahead of us and cautiously started walking away from the hill. I began to realize that Harold and I had just experienced a major transition in our lives. With God's help, we had shared an experience together that would last a lifetime. We had defeated death, God had won, and if we chose, He could use us once more.

"It wasn't long until we were deep in the jungle. The smell of rotting flesh still hung in the air but was now less offensive. The tension was high as we prayed that the NVA had had enough and would leave us alone. The heat and humidity hung in the air almost visibly. It was like walking through a steam bath wrapped in a hot towel. Our fatigues were soaked with sweat, turning them black. There was no relief from the heat, no breeze blew to cool us.

"We worked our way deeper into the twilight of the jungle. Occasionally patches of sunlight could be seen where there were tiny breaks in the thick canopy a hundred feet above. The deeper we went, the dimmer it became until we were in a world of perpetual twilight. The jungle thinned abruptly, the broad-leafed plants and lacy ferns giving way to thick grass several feet tall.

"We walked alone in single file with only our thoughts of the past five days. Memories of dead NVA left rotting on the jungle floor and of our friends who were wounded, never to be the same again, and of our friends who died there.

After an hour or so, the pace began to take its toll on us and we began to slow down. We halted and fanned out in a rough circle. We hadn't been followed and it appeared the enemy was going to leave us alone. The tepid water in my canteen tasted good, even with the halazone tablets in it. The insects attracted by the sweat darted at our eyes and buzzed around our ears. After a few minutes, the monkeys began their usual chatter and the birds squawked. These were good signs. We could rest easier because we were alone.

"Half an hour later, we saddled up and moved out once more. The point and flank security cautiously set out and we followed. In a few minutes, we topped over the crest of a small hill and down into the valley where a stream flowed. The ground turned marshy and wet, and the water felt cool and refreshing as we crossed the small stream. For once I wished it would have been deeper and we had time for a bath. Harold had been telling me a bath would do us both a world of good.

"We walked most of the day and then entered an old deserted village just before sundown. At the far end of this village was a piece of land sticking out into a deep rugged valley like a finger pointing west. On this finger of land, we found Charlie Company waiting for us.

"A perimeter had already been formed and we were to spend the night with them. On the three sides of this finger was steep shale, and the land was covered with giant teak trees. At the end of the finger was a log platform, which they had built to be used as a landing pad for choppers. The Hueys would enter the valley and touch down on this pad one at a time, their rotor blades coming very close to the trees. When they were ready to take-off, they would have to lift off slowly, turn around, and leave the same way they had entered.

"Charlie Company had also been in contact the past few days and this landing pad was built out of a desperate need for resupply and evacuating the dead and wounded. The two engineers that traveled with them had performed an almost impossible task. With the help of Charlie Company, they had built this platform by hand. The logs were huge and it was built out over the side of a steep hill. One person had been killed when a tree fell on him.

"To get to this finger of land, we had to cross over an open area about thirty feet wide and a hundred feet long. They had positioned their two machine guns at this point to keep the enemy from entering. The village was deserted but some of the animals were still there. It appeared to have been a Montagnard village and the people had fled.

"Throughout the night, the enemy would sneak through the village to get as close as possible to Charlie Company. As they came, the chickens and pigs would become frightened and start making noise. Because of this they had known the NVA were getting close. They had been able to repulse every attack and, like the enemy that had been trying to get at us, they too had fled back into Cambodia.

"As we entered the perimeter, I saw Ruben sitting in one of the positions. It was good seeing him. We all had been so close during our stay at Ft. Lewis and when we arrived in Vietnam we had become scattered in separate units. Out of our group I was only around Corky while we were in the field. Ruben looked as tired as I felt. The walk had been filled with stress and the humidity had been draining. At least now the guard duty would be shared between our two companies, and most everyone could get some much-needed rest.

"I looked at the luminous dial of my watch to see what time it was. It was still too early to get up, so I lay in silence listening to the nocturnal noises around me. They were safe and comforting sounds to hear. Soon dawn would be breaking, and the blackness would be turning to shades of grey. I looked to my left and saw the faint outline of the next position and could make out a dark lump of the person's head. I let my eyes wander over the jungle, listening to the light rustling of leaves as a breeze blew through. Soon I could pick out individual trees and bushes, as the jungle became light shades of grey instead of black. Patches of mist drifted up from the valley below and the sky became a golden ball of orange. Another humid day was about to be born. All of us inside that perimeter had experienced something new and tragic over the past five days. I doubt if there were very many who had enjoyed the violence that had and still did surround us.

"Years have passed since the late afternoon in 1967 when I walked into the McCord Air Force Base waiting room and saw my family waiting for me. I never had to experience the hostility many returning soldiers went through. I was never called baby killer or spit on, but I watched on television as this happened to others.

"Both my Mom and Dad have passed away now and my sister and I are senior citizens. My daughters are adults and I have grandkids in their twenties. One would think my Vietnam experience would be a fading memory, but I can honestly say that I have thought of Vietnam every day since my return. The nightmares ended many years ago and with the VA's help I now get a good night's sleep.

"My last job was as a therapist with the VA helping Vietnam Vets who were diagnosed with combat related posttraumatic stress disorder. This was the most rewarding job I ever had. I have stayed in contact with several of the medics I trained with. Sadly, Harold Stenseth and I attended the memorial service for Frank 'Corky' Colburn after his death from cancer, caused by Agent Orange. Each of us have been diagnosed with PTSD and either have cancer or type ll diabetes, also caused by Agent Orange. Every October I've thought of my first combat.

"I was a medic attached to Alpha Company 2/8th Infantry. My first combat was towards the end of October 1966 when I was the medic that came with my platoon Sergeant, the LT and seven others to reinforce Bravo Company who was hit and surrounded on a small hill. The first night I was there we were hit around 9:00 pm. I was in a foxhole with the Sergeant and LT half way up the hill when my first call for a medic came just moments after hell broke loose. It came from down in front of us.

"I jumped out of the hole and crawled down the hill to the perimeter and asked who called for a medic and the guy pointed out in front of us to a body laying very close to the jungle. The guy had been one of three who were on a listening post. One guy made it inside the perimeter, the one guy out in front of us and the other guy died at the LP.

"I ran out to the guy and knelt beside him. He was laying on his stomach and I could see in the moonlight a blood stain on his hip. I ask him if he was hit anywhere else and he said, 'Get down they're right behind us.' I gave him a shot of morphine and ran back to the perimeter and said that I needed help and a guy from Bravo Company jumped up and we ran out and carried the wounded back inside the perimeter. It is a miracle we were not KIA.

"I am a Christian and was one of the medics who never carried a weapon. Those of you who were in Bravo Company will remember that most of the medics in your company also never carried a weapon."

Medical supply support for the U.S. Army on active duty in Vietnam was excellent. It may have been easy to reproach the U.S. Army on many levels, but when it came to the medical services, they were second to none in Vietnam.

By the 1960s new methods had been devised to deal with new types of battlefield trauma, such as those inflicted by mines, high velocity missiles, and Vietnam style IEDs known back then as booby traps. Terrain factored significantly in this conflict as many wounded soldiers had to be extracted from difficult locations such as jungles and paddy fields or along waterways. Bell "Huey" helicopters were in abundance and usually available to evacuate casualties to medical facilities before the inflicted wound deteriorated beyond help.

Many factors contributed to the low mortality rate of casualties, such as rapid evacuation availability of whole blood, well-established forward hospitals, advanced surgical techniques, and improved medical management. Blood packaged in styrofoam containers, which allowed storage between forty-eight and seventy-two hours in the field, could be placed in the forward area in anticipation of casualties. Most forward hospitals in Vietnam even had air conditioning to neutralize the extreme heat, dust, and humidity and allow the use of state-of-the-art medical equipment.

Mary "Edie" Meeks was a U.S. Army Nurse, 3rd Field Hospital in Saigon. From July 1968 to January 1969 and from January to July 1969, she was stationed at the 71st Evac Hospital in Pleiku. This is her story in her own words.

"Enlistment: It was February 1968, they were quite surprised when I walked into the recruitment station and I said I was a nurse and I wanted to go to Vietnam. I signed up to go to Vietnam. We went to basic training in San Antonio, Texas, what we were taught was how to do traches, or tracheotomies on live animals, and this was because if things got so busy that they needed to put you up a slot, you'd be able to do what you needed to do. You'd have some idea of how to do it. It was kind of schizophrenic, basic training was, I went there because I wanted to take care of people. I wanted to take care of the soldiers. I joined mainly because my brother was drafted and he joined the Marines and at that time, I knew what it was like, if a nurse didn't want to be some place, but I figured I knew how to do this kind of nursing, I can go and I will want to be there. In case my brother was hurt, I would want someone to be there who wanted to be there. That was why I joined the Army.

"Army Training: You are taught how to save lives and you're taught all of the injuries that can happen. But then you have Colonels come in and tell you about the kill power of this weapon and that weapon, and he was almost drooling with joy over the power of these. Same with the Agent Orange. I'm sitting there thinking this is a crazy. But I was there to do a job that was different than what the Colonels were doing. It was 8 weeks of training and I met some great people there and they came from all over the country and all different ages and we didn't have men in our class, all females. A lot of them did not want to go to Vietnam.

"I went to Fort Ord, California for three months, and worked in an orthopedic ward. Where all we had were guys who came back from Vietnam and that was a huge basic training area. That was where I met my future husband. Then after three months there I went to San Francisco and then they sent me to Vietnam, which was also quite bizarre. You go from America, and you land in this country where everything is totally different and the mindset is totally different. You're told, if you stay in Saigon, don't kick the cans; they put explosives in the cans.

"3rd Field Hospital: I worked in intensive care in the 3rd Field Hospital. I remember one morning where we had 9 guys come in, they had been standing on a corner waiting for a bus, and somebody drove by on a little motorcycle and threw something that exploded. Luckily none of them died but you couldn't trust anyone. I remember we had a ward clerk he was a nice guy. One morning, I asked where our ward clerk was, and I was told that he was killed the night before and that he was VC. He was in a skirmish with our guys and got killed. You just never knew. Everyone seemed to be really nice but one of the difficulties of nursing there was when you would get a Vietnamese patient, now usually he was a prisoner. They wanted to stabilize him so that they could interview him. The mind thought immediately was "why do I have to waste my time on this guy, he's the enemy, and I need my time to take care of my guys." That was really an interesting ethical thing for me. I had to really think it through. You were taught as a nurse that you take care of the patient and take care of them equally. You were to give this person the same kind of care you would give anybody else. I had to really think of the thoughts in order to get through that.

"For me one of the most difficult things was the ages of these kids that we took care of, the average age was between 18 and 23 and those were the ages of my two brothers, they were both younger than I. In an Emergency Room, everything makes sense, it all makes sense, over there nothing made sense. These were perfectly healthy young men who came in blown to bits. As you're going on, you are wondering more and more why. They didn't seem to be allowing them to win. Even the guys would say that, 'They aren't letting us win.' The United States had one way to fight a war, there were rules to fighting the war, the North Vietnamese didn't have any rules and the guys hands were tied. It was kind of an unfair war produced by our government by micromanaging.

"By October of that year I was so filled with rage at our government, but also at the Army. I thought when you join the Army, the Army takes care of its own. These are citizen soldiers, they aren't mercenaries, they're citizens that have been asked to do something for the government and they're doing it. And yet they just seemed to be throwing these guys away. So 2,000 got hit, bring 2,000 more over it didn't seem to matter. And yet being the nurse, I knew these kids had families that were waiting at home for them. One of the toughest things for me, and I still get choked up about it, and this was the one that really haunted me, it opened the door into being in Vietnam. He was 19, he was from a farm in Kansas and he had a terrible abdominal injury. We had a lot of those, and chest wounds because the guys didn't wear their flak jackets cause they were 40 pounds. This kid got a letter from his mom and he asked me to read him the letter and I said sure. The mother said, "Oh your Dad and the family dog just came in from doing some pheasant hunting down on their farm' and talked about what was happening in town and people that they knew and at the very end she said 'we're so proud of you son,' and three days later he died.

"For me that was really the epitome of the difference between being the General who is just sending numbers and being the nurse who is taking care of a person. Because every one of those kids that came by, you knew had a family that was waiting for them, or a girlfriend or a wife. We had one guy come in one night, he was one of six and it was about 11 o'clock at night and we heard we would be getting this group of casualties and some of them went to surgery right away and some of them we stabilized. One of them was the Captain of this group of guys and the other guys who were not injured all came to the hospital, they all came with them. They kept asking about the Captain because he was just the most wonderful man. He died, he had a heart attack because his wounds were so bad, he died and he was 26 and he had three kids. You were sitting there saying this was the best of the best. These guys loved him, trusted him, and the government threw him away. The Army threw him way. So for me that was really, really difficult.

"There was no place you could put your rage, so what you did was you just shut down. You couldn't keep feeling because it was too overwhelming and because every time those guys would come in they were my brother. And to see my brothers are worth something, they're really great guys and so were these young men. So that was really really tough. You just shut down and you kept doing your job because you couldn't process, we were 12 hours a day, six days a week, minimum. Somebody said, did you go back and talk about it, and that was the last thing you wanted to do. Plus, you didn't have time, you had to go to sleep before you had to get up and work the next 12 hours. We never discussed anything like that, my roommate, Judy, from Saigon, she also worked in intensive care and we never talked about our patients. That was an interesting thing about Judy, I came back to the States after my tour was over and Judy called me and she was going to be getting married and then everybody's life went on. I never contacted anybody except Diane Carlson Evans.

"The dedication of the Women's Memorial was coming up and I could not remember Judy's name. Finally, I got to Washington at the hotel we were all staying in, and on the bulletin board there was a little piece of paper that said 'Edie if you're here, I'm in room so-so, Judy.' I thought 'Oh my God, that was her name.' So here was a gal I lived with for 6 months and went through hell together but then luckily enough the psychiatrist I went to said that wasn't uncommon forgetting things and parts of it.

"My brother, Tom was drafted and decided to go into the Marine Corps, at that time both of us lived in Los Angeles. When I joined the Army and I wrote him and I said, 'This is wonderful, I joined the Army and you know if anything happens to you.' And he said, 'Well Edie, that's wonderful, but the Navy takes care of the Marines.' I think he was relieved that his sister wouldn't be there in case something was to happen. What was really funny, I went down to visit him before I went over to Vietnam, and he was stationed at Camp Pendelton. They said, Go and ask for Gunnery Sergeant so and so, and he'll know where he is. Not even knowing what a Gunnery Sergeant was. So I asked for this gunnery sergeant and this guy turns around and he has a glass eyeball with the Marine Corps emblem on it. And I thought well this is dedication. I was talking to my brother about it and he said, he also has an eyeball with an American flag on it. What was interesting about being down there at that time, there were very few Marine Corps female officer was a surprise. Tom said, 'I like this,' cause he was a PFC, 'I like walking around and people have to salute you.' So Tom went places, Tom has never talked about with me, ever.

"My brother Charlie, signed up at the draft board as everybody does, but he was arrested for war protesting and somebody said to me, 'How did you feel about that?' and I said 'I knew my brother loved me but he hated the war.' He later told me if he had been drafted he would have gone. It wasn't that he wasn't going to do what he was supposed to do as a citizen, but he really needed to state that he didn't believe in the war. So that's what happened to my brothers.

"We didn't take of too many of the Marines, a lot of them they were flown out to Navy ships and more out on the coast, Pleiku was in the central Highlands near Laos, there was a big air force base near out hospital. Although I do have to say that one time I went to where the officers met where you were supposed to relax. There was a Marine Major and he had had a lot to drink and he was feeling really sad about the fact that this was his third tour in Vietnam and he still didn't have a Purple Heart. And for me being the nurse taking care of all these Purple Heart recipients it was, again, it's that kinda schizophrenic kind of thought process that you are dealing with, the whole mess of the services especially if you are caregiver, and your whole thing is to preserve life. One thing I did, I know that their motto is 'Preserve the fighting strength,' that was the last thing I wanted do, I wanted to preserve them so they could go home.

"But many of them, if for instance they had malaria and they would come to us in Pleikeu, a lot of the guys there, that they'd get better and be sent back. It was really crazy.

"When I first got to Saigon, I had been dating this guy, Bill, who I eventually married. And he was stationed in Saigon and his specialty was, he was a MSC officer, Medical Service Core, and his specialty was computers.

"They were computerizing all of the supplies going in and going out the country. When I first got there, he said, 'Let's go out to dinner,' after working 12 hours a day with these guys who had been blown to pieces. I said ok, because what did I know. But Saigon at that time still had five-star restaurants still from the French. You would go this fancy place and eat a fancy meal and after doing that twice, I said to him, 'I can't see you anymore, it's just too strange, it's too out of body, kind of.' So your whole life was based around the people in your unit, at least for us it was, because we were very tight in that we had to trust each other.

You could hang blood, if you found that the hemoglobin was way down, and you would trust that the doctor would back you on that, because he knew you. And you trust the Corpsmen, the Corpsmen were fabulous.

"I remember one night, the same night when the six guys were coming in who had been blown up and the Captain had died. There was usually two RNs on, half one side was intensive care, the other half was recovery room, once they stabilized for recovery room and once they would be shifted to the intensive care unit. But the gal who was supposed to be with me was still off on R & R so they didn't make it back. It wasn't that bad, we had maybe three on the intensive care side and maybe two on recovery room. Then we heard we were going to be getting these six that were in bad shape, and I told one of the Corpsman that they were in charge of the intensive care unit, tell me if somebody needs a medication but you're going to take vitals and going to do everything for them. The Corpsmen, as the night wore on, just stopped by to see what was happening and then went to work.

"They had worked a 12-hour shift many of them, but they all just pitched in and they kept coming in the door and pitching in. It was that kind of teamwork that you very seldom find in regular life and that was one of the things that the guys found difficult, and I found difficult too. After having such a tight-knit group that works so well together, coming back there isn't that anywhere. If these guys were out in the field, they depended on each other for their lives and then you come back here and there's nobody you can trust like that. The teamwork, I think it was because we were all in it for one thing, to keep these guys alive. Whereas nursing stateside the teamwork doesn't necessarily exist, that's why I like the operating room I work in now and because in the OR you have to work as a team and so it's still that feeling of respect. You get to know the people so well, you read their minds, they read yours, which is really a little bit of what it was like over there.

"It wasn't until I was going to be going home, the nurses that were coming in country were saying as soon as your come off the plane, take your uniform off, you will not be accepted, take a dress or whatever you're going to wear and change in the ladies room as soon as you get off the plane. So that's what I did, I threw my uniform in the trash. It was my fatigues, my boots, put on a dress and went home.

Because from going from Vietnam, which I left in '69, and eight months later living in New York City, it took me a while to get used to that."[110]

Approximately twelve thousand helicopters saw action in Vietnam (all services), and it's estimated that forty thousand pilots served in the war. Of the 2.29 million U.S. military who served in Vietnam, one out of every ten became a casualty in some way or another. Fifty-eight thousand, one hundred sixty-nine were killed and 304,000 were wounded. Although the percentage of dead is similar to other wars, amputations or crippling wounds were 300 percent higher than in World War II. Veterans returning from the Vietnam War were seldom (if ever) lauded with ticker tape parades or brass bands. More often than not, and due to no fault of their own, they were jeered at, derided, and denigrated by the errant youth of a nation living comfortable lives in a democracy that so many had fought and died for.

This story of PFC White is archetypal of the harrowing experiences many medics endured in the Vietnam War. [111]

"As the medevac helicopter settled onto the landing pad beside the battalion aid station, the litter bearers rushed through the swirling downdraft to lift the stretchers from its floor. I had been alerted that Bravo Company had a wounded man on board and had hurried to await its arrival.

"As they removed the stretchers from the helicopter, a man slid off the chopper and limped along beside one of the stretchers as it was rushed into the aid tent. When I moved alongside to see who had been wounded, I saw the pale white face of Doug Muller, a good friend and squad leader in my former platoon. Two bullets from a sniper had ripped through Doug's back.

---

[110] https://oralhistory.rutgers.edu/images/PDFs/meeks_edie.pdf.

[111] Author Bob Babcock CEO of Deeds Publishing. Used with permission. https://www.deedspublishing.com/.

"The man limping along beside the stretcher was the platoon medic, PFC Julian White. Blood oozed from a hole in his boot where a bullet from the same sniper had hit him. Ignoring his own wound, he continued to care for Doug.

"The scene continued to develop as they carried another stretcher from the chopper into the aid tent. This one carried the NVA soldier who had shot Doug and PFC White. One of our men had shot him down from his perch high up in a tree. Still alive when he fell to the ground, he became a prisoner and had to be cared for.

"The doctors worked hurriedly over the two stretchers, assessing the damage, stabilizing the wounds, and preparing the men for evacuation to 18th Surgical Hospital back at Pleiku. PFC White stayed right by Sergeant Muller's side as the doctors worked to save him.

"Finally, someone noticed White's limp and the blood seeping from the wound. Over his objections, he was put on a stretcher and a medic started to care for him. While watching PFC White's obvious concern and caring for Doug Muller, I remembered an incident aboard the troop ship a few months earlier. PFC White had gone AWOL (Absent Without Leave) while we were at Fort Lewis. He had been gone for six weeks but had shown up, to everyone's surprise, the day before the ship left for Vietnam. He was placed under arrest and boarded the ship with us.

"I was assigned as the prosecuting officer to bring the charges against him at his court martial. In preparing for the case, I interviewed him to find out why he had gone AWOL. He was very courteous and honest as he explained his reasons.

"He had entered the Army as a conscientious objector. Since he would not carry a rifle, he had been sent to medic school. He had been wrestling with his value system throughout his time in the Army. He had no questions about his own unwillingness to kill another human being, but he could not bring himself to grips with even being a part of an Army that did. After much soul searching, he had decided he could not participate in such an organization and went AWOL. While gone, he had drifted up and down the West Coast trying to sort out his beliefs. Besides not believing in killing others, he was also a very patriotic American citizen.

His AWOL status bothered him as much as his unwillingness to participate with a killing machine. After six weeks of anguish, he had decided he could not live with himself as a deserter and had returned to Fort Lewis.

"He had committed himself to doing everything he could to help his fellow man without getting involved in direct conflict with the enemy.

"After hearing his absolutely honest and open confession, I spent long hours trying to decide logically and objectively how I would prosecute the case. I was convinced he had already gone through enough self-imposed punishment. He did not need to receive any more than the minimum allowable punishment from the Army. But, my job was to prosecute him. He had broken an Army law that had been enforced since the days of George Washington.

"As I presented the facts to the court martial board, I requested they treat him with leniency. His defense council, Lieutenant Bill Saling, explained the circumstances PFC White had dealt with. Bill's eloquently presented defense argument convinced the board they were dealing with a good soldier whose value system priorities were in major conflict. After a short deliberation, the board returned a verdict of guilty.

"They imposed a sentence of fourteen days confinement to quarters, a virtual non-sentence under the circumstances, since we were all confined to the quarters of the ship. We knew then we had a good soldier in PFC Julian White.

"He had spent the first half of his tour working in the battalion aid station and had joined my old platoon just after I had left it. All the reports I had gotten were that he was doing an outstanding job looking after the men's daily aches and pains.

"When the sniper hit Doug Muller, PFC White immediately jumped up from his covered position to go to Doug's aid. Bullets pounded the area around him as he worked on Doug's wounds. When hit in the foot, he did not slow down but continued to focus all his efforts and attention on taking care of the seriously wounded man, completely ignoring his own safety.

"My mind came back to the activity in the aid station. The men working on the NVA soldier stopped their activities and covered his head. He had died before they could save him. After Doug's wounds were stabilized, he was hurried out to another waiting medevac helicopter and transferred to the surgeons at 18th Surgical Hospital.

"PFC White's stretcher was loaded on the same chopper. My guess was PFC White again forgot his own wound and made sure Doug was properly cared for on the short flight. I took much care and pride in writing the recommendation to award PFC Julian White a Bronze Star for Valor for his actions. He was truly a sincere human being who cared greatly for his fellow man."

It was the first real media war that was filmed, recorded, and scrutinized by journalists and displayed on TV screens throughout the world. Peculiarly enough, news coverage was not subjected to government censorship. The veterans were in some cases ostracized by an ungrateful nation; they had done their duty and sacrificed their young years to serve a country that initially didn't want to know. At least they had the comfort of knowing that if they got wounded there was always the medevac teams on standby and ready to fly wherever the action was.

Medevac helicopters flew nearly five hundred thousand missions in Vietnam, airlifting nine hundred thousand patients (of whom almost one-half were Americans). The average time lapse between being wounded and reaching a hospital was usually less than one hour, and as a result, less than 1 percent of the casualties died of their wounds within the first twenty-four hours. This was mainly because of the talents of medevac physicians who opened surgical airways, performed thoracic needle decompressions and shock resuscitation en route to the allocated destination.

Between January 1965 and December 1970, 133,447 wounded were admitted to medical treatment facilities in Vietnam, 97,659 of which were admitted to hospitals. Apart from the medevac helicopters, the U.S. military had five separate companies and five detachments of ground ambulances at their disposal; however, the primary purpose for these vehicles was transporting casualties from the landing strip or LZ to the hospital facility. Sometimes they were used to transport patients to other hospitals, but this depended largely on how secure the chosen route was at the time.

Despite the effectiveness of medevac helicopters in Vietnam, they were frequently beset by the problem of finding suitable landing zones in proximity to the action. In the jungle and on steep terrain, it was often impossible to land the helicopter. Therefore in many cases, the wounded had to be moved to the nearest accessible site, but this entailed using personnel to physically carry the wounded from A to B. This only served to extend the waiting time and discomfort of the casualties. The solution to this problem was the Personnel Rescue Hoist, which was developed and improved to a reliable model by mid-1966.

Once the UH-1 helicopter was equipped with the necessary electrical system, the aircraft crew could quickly install or remove the hoist as required. The hoist itself consisted of a winch and cable on a boom that was extended out from the aircraft when it arrived over the rescue site. It was anchored to the floor and roof of the helicopter cabin, usually just inside the right-side door behind the pilot's seat. When the door was open, the hoist could be rotated on its support to position the cable and pulleys outside the aircraft, clear of the skids, so that the cable could be lowered to and raised from the ground. At the end of the cable was a ring and hook to which a Stokes litter, rigid litter, or forest penetrator could be attached. The cable could be lowered at the rate of 150 feet per minute and retracted at the rate of 120 feet per minute. A slight variation on the theme was the forest penetrator, a spring-loaded device that could penetrate dense foliage and opened to provide seats on which a casualty could be securely strapped in. This hoist was the preferred choice by the crews over the litter version because it was less likely to become entangled in the trees and foliage.

On a hoist mission, the medical corpsman or crew chief would use the hoist cable to lower a litter or harness to casualties below while the aircraft hovered. The crew chief would sometimes lower a medical corpsman with the device. Then the hoist would raise both the medic and the casualty to the helicopter. The standard hoist could lift up to six hundred pounds in one load and could lower a harness or litter about 250 feet below the aircraft. The only significant problem encountered by crew when they were using the hoist was that the helicopter became a "sitting duck" for enemy troops in the area while it was undertaking an extraction. In 1968, thirty-five aircrafts were by hit hostile fire while on hoist missions. That number increased to thirty-nine in 1969.

The term "Dustoff" was coined in Vietnam when it was chosen in 1963 from a codebook as the call sign for the 57th Medical Detachment. It evoked images of a Huey helicopter taking off from the dry and dusty Vietnam countryside and came to represent all medevac helicopter operations. The 57th Medical Detachment has the honor of being regarded as "The Original Dustoff."

Most air ambulances had qualified "flight surgeons" on board. They were qualified physicians who had received formal training in the specialized field of aviation medicine. They were usually attached to an aviation brigade, which was in turn supported by a medical detachment team that provided dispensary service. When the situation allowed, triage and primary care for the wounded could be performed en route by the flight surgeons. The helicopter was indeed fast and efficient but it was also vulnerable to ground attack. Heavy bombers in World War II often flew missions that could take hours, but within the duration of the mission they would only be vulnerable to enemy fire for between ten and twenty minutes. In contrast to that, helicopters in Vietnam were almost constantly exposed to hostile fire, even in their base camps.

The terrain may have been radically different but like WWI, Vietnam was a war of attrition where each side chipped away relentlessly at each other's units; however, success wasn't measured in territory gained. It was measured in body counts. Another similarity is in the many futile objectives (operations executed with courage, stoicism, and discipline but often of little or no avail). Vietnamese hills and valleys paid for in American blood were frequently abandoned and dismissed without explanation. It is, however, an irrefutable fact that U.S. casualties incurred in the Vietnam War received better and faster treatment than in any previous conflict. This was achieved because it was discovered early on in the war that relatively small numbers of helicopters had the capacity to evacuate larger numbers of patients to centrally located medical facilities much quicker than their predecessors.

The primary medevac helicopters in Vietnam were the UH-1 Huey, UH1-D, and UH-1H, but others were also employed for this purpose. When a request was made for a rapid response for casualty evacuation, the air ambulance crews that scrambled had sufficient basic medical training to enable them to perform accurate triage and evaluate a patient's condition. They would then recommend the most suitable destination and provide resuscitative care en route. Such professionalism and dedication was unprecedented.

One of the reasons medical units stationed in Vietnam were compelled to develop better proficiency and a certain degree of autonomy because the nearest offshore U.S. hospital was almost one thousand miles away at Clark Air Force Base in the Philippines. These extended distances, even with modern air transport, demanded a nominal degree of self-sufficiency to be able to operate in the combat operation zones. The standard of qualifications and proficiency exceeded what had been required of medical staffs in previous wars. During the Vietnam War, the U.S. military deployed a significantly higher ratio of medical to combat troops than had been used before in military operations.

Nurse Helen Eileen Hause served at 4162nd Air Force Hospital, 92nd Tactical Air Command Hospital, 6160th Air Force Hospital, 9th Aeromedical Evacuation Squadron, 820nd Medical Group and 81st Tactical Air Command Hospital. She recalled the following:

"I said to the chief nurse, you know, I'd like to go to Vietnam. And she said, 'So would every other nurse. I said, 'Okay. She said, 'Put your name on a list. The list is so long, you know, you don't have to worry about it. Well, I said somebody must have burned the list, because three months later, I had my orders to go to Tan Son Nhut. We had an 85-bed staging unit. The Army would bring in the wounded to the third field hospital, which was a big general hospital inside that, and take care of the guys, do their thing with them. And then they would bring them out to us. We would process them into the aerovac system. They would bring them in. We would keep them overnight, change their dressings, get them into pajamas, give them baths, feed them, and then board them on the plane the next day.

"And sometimes they would come in from the MASH units occasionally, directly from the MASH unit. These guys would still have the red clay of Vietnam on them, so we would, you know, do our thing with bathing and feeding and changing dressings. I just couldn't understand how humans could stand up to what those kids had just suffered and survived. It was amazing.

"I was proud of my sister nurses in the Army. One of the hospitals units got mortared, and some of the nurses were killed. I was terrified because at night you could hear mortar fire, and you could look up in the air, and see tracer fire from the gunships flying around. On January, the 2nd or 3rd when they had tipped my friend who was there. I was the day shift. We had bunk beds in our rooms. Our rooms were probably maybe 8 X 10. Not very big. But they put bunk beds in there, just in case some other female officers might need a space or the other flight nurses, MAC flight nurses, might need to hang out. Another nurse asked me 'Can I come down and sleep in your room when I get off duty?' And I said, 'Sure,' you know. 'It doesn't bother me. Sleep up in the top bunk.' I don't know why this happened. I don't understand what this happened or why she did that. My room was just down the hall from the stairs, but hers was on the other side of the building. At 2 o'clock in the morning, they started to mortar Tan Son Nhut. And if you have never heard mortar rounds, it sounded like thunder claps. So we threw the robes on, and down the steps we went. I got to the -- She was ahead of me. And I got to the end of the last step, and I tripped, and I spread-eagled out on the cement.

"Terrified. 'Boom, boom, boom,' you know. Flames. The night sky was lit up. Oh God. It was terrifying. You could hear the small-arms fire. It was awful. And I said the other 'hooch' next to us had sandbags around it, or they hadn't gotten to ours to put sandbags around it. So I said, 'We have got to get over to that 'hooch' and get behind those sandbags, to protect us from flying stuff.' And so we all got down. I picked myself up. I dove into this one other one gal's room that had four people in there already, and two were under the table, two were under the bed, and there was no room for me. So I said, 'We have got to go next door and get behind the sandbags.' It was mayhem. It was just absolute mayhem. But we did it. And we got over behind the sandbags, and my knees were just banging together. I was oh God so bothered. It was just 'clang, clang, clang.' Oh dear. After that first night, the mortar rounds would come in every other night so that was an interesting period of my life.

"Oh. The day I left there was the day I got up to Johnson Air Force Base, and there were the headlines that Martin Luther King had been shot. And I thought, 'Oh my God,' because my sister had died while I was in Vietnam, and I had come home. And a friend of mine was living in Detroit, and she said, 'Why don't you come up and stay in Detroit with me' after we dealt with my funeral, or my sister's arrangements. They were having a riot in Detroit, this horrible riot of 1967. And she lived in a penthouse. I was out on her deck, watching the people below, you know. There they were, the same armaments that they had in Vietnam. Twenty people had been killed. I said, you know, 'This is ridiculous. This is downtown Detroit, Michigan, and here these people are killing each other,' When I got to Japan, there were these headlines, I knew that I was going to have trouble getting home. So I got into San Francisco. And of course I had to fly out on commercial. And, you know, the Vietnam veterans weren't being treated very well so they said, 'Change your clothes and get into civilian clothes.' 'Okay.' And so then I landed in Detroit around 2 o'clock in the morning. And of course Wayne County was closed so I had to call my friend up. And I said, 'Can I come and stay with you?' Because my brother couldn't come to get me, because they wouldn't allow him to come up there. So I stayed with her for two days, and then my brother came and picked me up. And so that's how I got out of Vietnam."[112]

By the time the conflict came to an end, there were over five thousand American nurses working in Vietnam with an average age of 23.6. Sixty-one percent of those killed were younger than twenty-one years old. Eleven thousand four hundred and sixty five younger than twenty years old [113] The average age of male fatalities was 23.1 years. Despite the use of

---

[112] "Helen Eileen Hause," Experiencing War: Stories from the Veterans History Project (Library of Congress, October 26, 2011), https://memory.loc.gov/diglib/vhp-stories/loc.natlib.afc2001001.23490/.

[113] https://www.uswings.com/about-us-wings/vietnam-war-facts/.

the draft, two-thirds of the men who served in Vietnam were volunteers. These volunteers accounted for approximately 70 percent of those killed in Vietnam. In conclusion, the fall of Saigon happened on April 30, 1975, two years after the American military left Vietnam. The last American troops departed in their entirety on March 29, 1973. Just for the record, it's important to point out that it was the South Vietnamese who lost the war, not the Americans who fought it.

CHAPTER EIGHTEEN

Iraq and Afghanistan

The reason allied Army, Navy, and Air Force medical departments began to deploy to the Persian Gulf as part of a multinational effort called Operation Desert Shield was to provide this force was equipped with a full range of medical support. U.S. diplomats immediately began urging, pressing Saudi Arabia to admit American troops to deter possible further Iraqi aggression. Saudi Arabia was initially reluctant to invite Christians and female soldiers into a country that is revered by Muslims. Another item of contention was the displaying the Red Cross on hospitals in a Muslim country, although this was quickly approved. The U.S 12th Evacuation Hospital (at that time located in Germany) would be the first hospital to deploy to the Middle East. The 12th was earmarked to support VII Corps, but at that time it was woefully unprepared. The unit had half its nonmedical strength (administrative officers and nonmedical enlisted personnel), but no actual medical personnel at their disposal. To compensate for this, the 7th MEDCOM drew individual soldiers from other medical units and facilities in Europe. They even borrowed staff included enlisted medical personnel such as pharmacy technicians, operating room technicians, and licensed practical nurses, as well as maintenance personnel, especially senior noncommissioned officers and maintenance warrant officers.

General paranoia about the possible use of chemical weapons inspired Major General Michael Scotti, the commander of 7th MEDCOM, to initiate two particular training tasks for units preparing for deployment. The priority was focusing on how to handle the harsh desert environment without degrading their operations, and they had to fully prepare for the possible eventuality of Saddam's army using chemical WMDs (weapons of mass destruction). It's a well-recorded historical fact that no WMDs were ever found in Iraq.

In preparation for "Operation Desert Storm," U.S. Air Force planes and Navy ships moved to the area, along with Marine Corps units that used equipment already on site. Their challenge was to send a trained and equipped medical system more than seven thousand miles, to provide care for a population larger than that of Seattle (and dispersed over an area approximately one-fifth the size of the continental United States), and to prepare simultaneously for the expected continuous flow of mass casualties. Active U.S. military physicians, dentists, nurses, and other healthcare personnel from community hospitals and medical centers were quickly dispatched to serve in the battalions, brigades, divisions, ships, air wings, hospitals, and field medical units being deployed to the Persian Gulf.

The Coalition's main logistics port was an area outside the port of Dhahran. For two weeks the main body of the 12th was stationed there in a tent city. This time was used practically to organize the unit and integrate the newly-arrived medical staff with nonmedical personnel. The chief nurse was obliged to meet all the new nurses, learn their qualifications and experience, and then assign them an appropriate position. Arriving equipment was unloaded, missing items were secured, and transportation was arranged. It was "game on."

At 3:00 a.m. Baghdad time on January 17, 1991, Operation Desert Storm was unleashed with the intention of driving Saddam Hussein's Iraqi forces from Kuwait. The precursor to Desert Storm began as an intense bombing campaign that devastated Iraq's infrastructure and destroyed many military supply lines. The air campaign was quickly followed by a ground war that lasted one hundred hours, in which a vast international coalition led by five hundred thousand U.S. troops routed the world's fourth largest army. The "mother of all battles" predicted by Saddam Hussein didn't take long to deteriorate for the Iraq forces and become the mother of all retreats.

In the wake of the terrorist attacks on the United States that occurred September 11, 2001, U.S. military forces were mobilized and deployed to Afghanistan (Operation Enduring Freedom (OEF)) in 2001 and to Iraq (Operation Iraqi Freedom (OIF)) in 2003. These forces had at their disposal highly trained and specialized Army field medical units, such as the previously mentioned Mobile Army Surgical Hospital (M.A.S.H.), the Combat Support Hospital (CSH), and the Forward Surgical Team (FST), as well as equivalents that accompanied Air Force and Navy units. These medical teams became almost immediately familiar with the types of casualties, both military and civilian, caused by insurgent guerrilla warfare; however, thanks to advances in both civilian and military medicine more soldiers are surviving grievous wounds than in previous conflicts. One young doctor remembers all too well. He wrote, "The first incident that really struck me, was actually an incoming incident.

"Somehow we had gotten intel that there would be an attack on the base (FOB Warrior/Kirkuk Regional Airbase, KRAB). My company, a forward support medical company, basically a medical company designed to support an infantry brigade, was living out of an aircraft bunker that was about 100 meters from the actual wire (it was still strands of actual razor wire at that time, the Berm wouldn't be built until later). So they got us all up into the Aircraft bunker, and we were all packed in the back half where the Patient Hold section was. I was assigned to Pt Hold at the time (I would later transfer to Ambulance Platoon) so my area was chalk full of my company. Some were playing games some were just talking. We weren't really doing anything.

"Then I heard SPC Bear yell 'INCOMING!' then slam the wooden door to the Command Post. Everybody froze. I remember looking at Sgt Woolstenhulme, the psych tech attached to us. He started saying 'that's not funny, you can get in a lot of trouble.' Just then I heard the BANG. I can't really describe it. there was a quick swoosh and the bang wasn't like the typical explosion. We all hit the deck. Then we were hustled down to the pilot's quarters in the bottom of the bunker, which was the XO's room. We passed the actual motor lodged in the classroom wall. The rocket fuel was still in the air. After a few minutes down there they got us all out because there was fear that there might be another hit and we could be potentially trapped. So we were brought outside and our first sergeant's first thought was an accountability formation. About this point the entire city of Kirkuk erupted in happy fire. The CO ordered a defensive parameter and for the next half hour or so I was pointed back towards the rest of the FOB while the city erupted behind me. I was scared shitless. I almost shot at the EOD team that came to check out our rocket hit.

"After they called the All Clear, I sat down outside the aircraft bunker and thought 'fuck I need a cigarette.' I overheard the EOD guys talking to the CO, and they said that if it had gone off it likely would have killed everyone in the bunker. It was a dud that shattered on impact. Imagine that. After that moment the ever-present fear left me and I found my faith again. It doesn't mean I wouldn't get scared, but I had more faith that things would end how they should.

keep in mind that's the FIRST major thing that happened to me on my first tour.

"After PFC Andre Craig died on 25 June 2007, I felt guilty that I didn't really know the guy, so I decided to pick one guy in my platoon and get to know everything about them. The man I picked was PFC James Jacob 'Spanky' Harrelson. He was pockmarked by acne, soft-spoken and…well, kind of a private. There's just something about privates. they think they know a lot until they're proven they don't, and always seem to piss off their NCOs. he liked being called Spanky cuz he looked like the character on the little rascals which amazed me because I didn't think anyone else knew that show. He was from Alabama, had that drawl, and could have been called "trailer trash" by some, but he was genuinely the kindest young man I had ever met. Man. He was only 3 days past his

19th birthday when he was killed. He was a driver for 2-2, and his vehicle got hit by 3 155mm arty rounds buried underneath the vehicle. Some say he was killed instantly. Another person said they heard him screaming. I had nightmares about that for years.

"The vehicle burned furiously. The rounds cooking off. It's like the popcorn from hell. Thousands of rounds. You could tell 5.56, 7.62, .50 and shotgun rounds. I was treating four men on the berm. honestly, this is one of those days I would really have to expand on, a lot, because there's a clear before and after. Anyway, after Spanky died, I went into a funk, and I tried not to get close to anyone.

"There's an incident, which may be barracks rumor or may actually have happened, for obvious reasons I can neither confirm nor deny they actually happened.

"'Iraq, 2004 in AO North on a little FOB that once belonged to one of Sadam's 'face cards.'

"There is an Aid station that has a problem. The problem is a Commo NCO that they technically need to fill radios and maintain the nets they listen to for MEDQRF, but is just about the most obnoxious ass ever. At the time when troops wanted to watch movies, they would use portable DVD players that had 6″ screens and very small speakers. Someone talking constantly makes it hard to hear. Also, someone farting the most atrocious gas imaginable and loudly eating all the junk food you've managed to scrounge through "connections" will get on anyone's nerves.

"One day a young bright eye bushy-tailed medic was having a M*A*S*H marathon while on standby and there was a plotline about this drug that turns a Marine bowler's urine blue. This young medic turns to the provider and says:

"'There isn't really a pill that turns your urine blue is there sir?'

"'What, methlin Blue? Oh yeah, it's used to diagnose certain kidney issues.'

"'Really?'

"'Oh yeah.'

"'Is it dangerous?'

"'[Laugh] no.'

"'Do we have any?'

"[Doctor's face drops all mirth] 'Why?'

"'Oh I was just curious.'

"[Doctor gives suspicious look, but no more is said on the subject]

"Fast forward two weeks while this young Medic is on a LogPac back to the brigade headquarters he stops into the main Class VIII supply shop for the brigade. He hands a list of medications his aid station needs and somewhere in the list is the vaunted Methylene Blue. The clerk takes the list and disappears for a while. The medic thinks about the newly arrived Burger King trailer and how he would literally kill for a whopper. He thinks how long it's been since he's had a good burger, and how he won't get one this LogPac because he's got to fix his M-998 Field Litter Ambulance. The clerk is gone for a long time. The medic starts to worry. Finally, the clerk shows up and says:

"'Sorry for the wait, I had to dig around for this one. Here are your meds.'

"Low and behold, they, in fact, had it. Methylin Blue. And since he's not getting any controlled substances...he doesn't have to sign for it. The medic may have grinned evilly here. Sources are conflicting.

"The medic took these meds, fixed his FLA, and tragically, missed out on Burger King.

"Another week passes. The young medic has really gotten into Stargate SG-1 and the commo NCO is getting on his very last nerve. The last straw is a nostril burning fart that causes the medic to flee during the climax of an episode. The NCO gets up to pee and the young medic takes his chance. Into the Diet Coke goes the Methylin Blue.

"NCO returns and drinks it. Time passes. Another diet coke is had. The NCO goes to the bathroom again.

"A high pitched girlish scream comes from the bathroom. The NCO runs into the aid station. Pants around his ankles.

"'MY GOD DAMN PISS IS BLUE!' he screams.

"The medic gets wide eyed and says, 'Wow. That sounds bad. I'm going to go get the doctor.'

"He doesn't get far. Everton in the aid station had heard it and came running. The Doctor got a suspicious look on his face immediately when the young medic said, 'Sir, it appears Sgt [name redacted]'s urine is blue.'

"'WHAT THE HELL IS GOING ON HERE?' The NCOIC of the aid station roared. The young medic was at this point fighting a valiant effort not to laugh.

"'Sergeant, it appears that sergeant [name redacted]'s urine has turned blue, and he is quite alarmed.'

"There are some things that are just so odd that their brain short circuits and they simply say "what?" by all accounts the NCOIC did that.

"The doctor and the NCOIC then proceed to "treat" the patient. The medic then proceeded to laugh so hard he thought he was going to break a rib. The medic reportedly did many push ups and nearly had the book thrown at him. The commo NCO kept his appearances in the Aid Station to a minimum.

"One thing that sticks out. How much your perception changes. Before the things that were intolerable now are nearly inconvenient. The things that would have sent me into a rage are only annoying. Conversely, things that I thought were really important are trivial. People say 'freedom isn't free.' I know in violent gory detail the price of freedom. How easy it is to cause people to live in fear. I know how lucky the West and Americans, in particular, have it. I've seen how bad it gets."[114]

At the time of writing, America—supported by the United Kingdom and other NATO allies—has been continuously involved in a war for well over a decade. A total of about 2.5 million Americans, roughly three-quarters of 1 percent, have served in Iraq or Afghanistan at some point in the post 9/11 years (many of them more than once). The main distinction in these recent conflicts is that more women have assumed front line combat duties than in any previous wars. The extent of female service members' involvement in OEF and OIF, in terms of both the number of women deployed and the scope of their involvement, is unprecedented. In 2010 the U.S. Army Special Operations Command

---

[114] Author interview. Real name withheld.

created a pilot program to put women on the battlefield in Afghanistan and in January 2016, the armed services lifted a controversial ban on women serving in positions of direct combat. Since then, women soldiers have patrolled the streets of Fallujah and Kandahar. They have driven in convoys on desert roads and mountain passes; they have deployed with Special Forces in Afghanistan on cultural support teams; they have scrambled into the cockpits of fighter jets and crawled out of the bloody rubble caused by IED explosions. They have become an integral part of all military operations.

One person who experienced Iraq firsthand was Corrine Lynn Schurz from Easton, Pennsylvania. Her interview has a very contemporary, candid feel to it, and confronts one of the many issues facing today's military. Being openly gay, she was eager to serve her country and learn a useful life skill, so she enlisted in the United States Army as a Radiology Specialist. She began training as a Medical Specialist (Combat Medic) and went on to become an X-Ray Specialist. After AIT (Advanced Individual Training) she was stationed in West Germany. While there she earned the Expert Field Medical Badge and was promoted to Specialist 5. After returning to the United States, she joined the U.S. Army Reserve and spent the next nineteen years as an actively drilling reservist in the numerous medical units that were staffed by the Reservists drilling in Grand Rapids, Michigan, and ending with the 323rd Combat Support Hospital and the 322nd Medical Company based in Southfield, Michigan. During her time as a drilling reservist, Schurz was promoted to Sergeant First Class. She graduated from Nursing School and was commissioned as a Second Lieutenant in June 2003.

First LT. Schurz deployed with the 325th Combat Support Hospital to COB Speicher, outside Tikrit, Iraq, where she served as a Medical-Surgical Nurse caring for injured and sick Americans, Iraqis, Coalition Forces, and Third Country Nationals (working as contractors). A Combat Support Hospital (CSH) has the job of stabilizing the patient and providing specialized treatment within a combat zone. Patients who couldn't be returned to duty were evacuated to hospitals in U.S. military bases in Europe. An active CSH provided up to 248 beds and was capable of providing general, orthopedic, thoracic, vascular, urological, and gyne-cological surgery. The CSH has extensive laboratory capabilities: X-ray, ultrasound scan, CT scan, blood bank, and physiotherapy.

While deployed, First LT. Schurz received the Army Commendation Medal. She ended her twenty-eight-year military career "honorably" on June 29, 2008, as a result of President Clinton's "Don't Ask, Don't Tell" policy. Don't ask, don't tell (DADT) is the term commonly used for the policy restricting United States military personnel from efforts to discriminate or harass closeted homosexual or bisexual service members or applicants while barring those who are openly gay, lesbian, or bisexual from military service. Schurz continues to live with her loving partner, soon to be spouse, of ten years.

"I joined the Army in May of 1980 and went to basic training in July of that year. I went to Fort Leonard Wood, Missouri, where--well, Missouri, it was a pretty hot summer. I'm sure we've had hotter since, but Missouri was known for having the most deaths from the heat shortly before I started there. I wanted a challenge. I am a lesbian and have al-ways been a lesbian, and so part of it was which branch of service was less likely to care or toss me out because of being a lesbian. The Marines don't have a medical field, and that's where I wanted to go because I figured--for a couple of reasons. One, I did not think that the--it was likely that the medical field would ask me to do things that were, that violated my personal code of ethics.

"My memory of Iraq. Iraqi dust and the smell of Iraqi dust just because there's not enough moisture to have a lot of anything else. The Hesco barriers that were basically big sandbags that made walls so we were safer. Just having to walk through the dust and the river rock that they put to make sure that when there was rain, because basically there was this layer of dust and then there was rock, bedrock kind of stuff un-derneath you. You know, the river rock was to keep you above the water when the puddles formed because, yes, it would rain, it just didn't have anywhere to go when it did. I was there from August till June, so I didn't get the heat of the summer, thank God, but we did get whatever the rainy season of winter was called.

"The only time they let me leave post was I took a Chinook ride as part of an exercise on how to load and unload litters, you know, casualties. So I was pretending to be a casualty. So I got loaded on. I got to see, you know, what the flight was like and then got off, and then when I left to go on pass to Kuwait for my four days of R and R. So, you know, our hospital commander is like you are not going to leave, we are not going to lose any of you, you will not leave the gate.

"My duties were the following. I worked in the intermediate care ward on the night shift, so we primarily took care of--so, basically I was a medical/surgical nurse. We basically took care of anybody that was sick because medical stuff was sort of, medical assets were divided up. We had the medical assets, so if there were women that were in the rest of the theatre that needed any of those services which were GYN, not really OB because that wasn't on the list but, you know, so if somebody had a female problem, they came to us. So we took care of folks that were sick. There were soldiers that could go back to duty. We took care of folks that were injured, that way usually they got, if they were American they got Evac'd. If they were coalition forces they got Evac'd. We took care of third country nationals that were mostly working as contractors, and we took care of Iraqis, the police, the Army and civilians that got injured so. We did have a couple of mass casualties, so we got to take care of them. You know, war is pretty violent and doesn't make a lot of sense most of the time.

"I think that the thing that moved me most was if we had folks that were in custody, I remember that there was a prisoner that was, you know, he was probably a teenager, and my understanding of Iraqi culture is that there can be a lot of innocence in making decisions. So here is this young kid. You know, he's probably, I don't know, somewhere between 17 and 19. He certainly is still single, he's still living with his mom kind of guy, and he is terrified because he is getting ready, once he is healthy enough, he is going to go to wherever we're detaining folks, and so he had another young soldier that was guarding him, and, you know, the heart that was still there, you know, the kid is sharing his IPod with him. But when he was ready, they were ready to put him on the aircraft to transfer him to detention, and he was like no, I'm sure I'm sick about something else, there is something else wrong with me. I have to be evaluated again, I can't go, and that was just heart-breaking, you know. So, the collateral damage, you know, the little baby that, you know, we took care of. You know, it's just, it's a violent thing, and it's not really always for the best reasons, you know. It's great when you got to protect yourself, but going after the bad guy can be bad.

"I found support in my spiritual group. I do not participate in revealed religion, so I am not part of the Abrahamic tradition. So, I found camaraderie largely from those that also follow the older faiths. And they were not from my unit, they were just the folks that were stationed on post, and so it was a little bit more eclectic of a group of people. And I deployed with the 325th Combat Support Hospital out of Independence, Missouri and there were something like 35 different states represented in my unit, and I deployed with two other people that I knew beforehand. So, we didn't have a lot of, oh, you know, I just, I always kind of felt like the outlier.

"I became friends with Major Martha Ryan from Massachusetts; Captain Leslie Cooper from Kansas City, I can't say which side of the state, which side of the river; Specialist Kyle Ellis from the 101st Airborne Division, which is really air. Those were probably my primaries. I stayed in touch with my family and friends back home through Skype and phone calls, and mostly it was just my partner, Elle, that I stayed in contact with, yeah. I called my mother every now and then.

"While I was deployed somebody felt uncomfortable with me. This somebody was a captain who was a nurse anesthetist who was scared of her shadow. That started out as a sexual harassment investigation, and according to my hospital commander, Colonel Hale, when he explained it to me he had informed his higher headquarters, the medical brigade, that he was having a sexual harassment investigation, and they said no, no, it's not a sexual harassment investigation, it's a Don't Ask, Don't Tell investigation, and hopefully anybody that's listening to this now, Don't Ask, Don't Tell has been in the history books for so long that you don't know what it is. So Don't Ask, Don't Tell was signed into law by President

Clinton in like 1996, and it basically said we won't ask you about whether you're a homosexual or behaving like one and you won't tell us.

"So that investigation was not decided in my favor. So, I was honorably discharged after my return home with my unit. So nobody lost a day of my performing with my unit as a nurse. I was given an end of tour Army Commendation Medal because I had earned it like everyone else, but what I got was an honorable discharge to go with it. So, after 28 years of active and reserve service, I will get a retirement when I turn 60, but I was discharged, and during that four months of investigation and the processing of everything that had to happen because I was a reservist who had already earned her retirement, nobody in the command of the theatre of Iraq could authorize my discharge, the Department of the Army had to say, yeah, you can discharge her. So, that was a very isolating experience because I was told that I wasn't allowed to discuss it with anyone. Our mental health services said you have to go to combat stress if you need to talk to somebody. I'm like, one, I don't know where that is; two, I'm working nights, and three, you know, there's no way. I'm going to go find some other folks to figure out what's what.

"Inevitably people found out because they had to collect evidence, quote unquote, of my telling because they didn't find any behavior that was inappropriate. One of the folks that wrote a statement against me said, well, two of them actually said, and she's my friend, which is pretty much the last time you can say that about somebody when you're kind of betraying them by writing this statement. One of them was like, oh, yeah, she gave me a hug. Well, a hug is not inappropriate support of somebody after they've just shared that, you know, I went home and my husband, is expressing infidelity towards me, and so I'm being supportive in giving you a hug, but somehow because I'm a lesbian that makes it a lesbian act. No! But people have craziness. The inappropriateness in this or that was that person was engaged in an extramarital affair with an enlisted person as an officer and nothing happened to them, but according to the Uniform Code of Military Justice it was certainly possible to bring charges against her, but no, just me after all that time, no problem. It was a problem for me, just so you know.

"I went back to my nursing job and worked it until we parted ways. I worked in corrections nursing for a while, and currently I am not employable as far as the VA is concerned, so I am totally and permanently disabled, and thank you for your efforts on my behalf for that. I served with some of those women that were the first graduating class of West Point. I certainly have served with many women that have honored themselves, and many of them, certainly from my perspective, were lesbian, not all, and sexual orientation doesn't make a good or bad soldier one way or the other, whichever way we are in it, but clearly for my identity it's been important to find my sisters in common. I think that lesbians in the service haven't really been recognized because we, just as gay men, had to be under the radar. So coming out to me is important in the process. So, since the Army had already gotten it, we're there."[115]

Almost 90 percent of combat medics assigned with line units participated in combat patrols, and most of those experienced some type of hostile incoming fire. Roughly a third witnessed someone from their unit or an ally being seriously wounded or killed, or enemy troops being seriously wounded or killed. The signature wounds of returning Iraq and Afghanistan war veterans are represented by the dual conditions of post-traumatic stress disorder (PTSD) and traumatic brain injury (TBI). Anger and aggression can be symptoms of both conditions.

The military history of Afghanistan is a long and bitter legacy. Many historians have often accurately referred to Afghanistan as the "graveyard of empires." Over two thousand years ago Alexander the Great experienced the fighting in the northeast. For him and his army it was a long and bloody war of guerrilla actions and sieges, and Alexander would spend the better part of three exhausting years attempting to subjugate the recalcitrant peoples of the distant *satrapies* of the region. He would inevitably fail. The British invasion of 1839 initially produced a stunning victory for the empirical army, but this was quickly followed by a stunning defeat that was consequently followed by a second victory. In

---

[115] Amy Pocan, "Interview with Corrine Schurz," Veterans History Project (Library of Congress, November 7, 2014), http://memory.loc.gov/diglib/vhp/story/loc. natlib.afc2001001.97568/transcript?ID=sr0001.

1878, the British invaded again. Though they suffered a major defeat at Maiwand, their main army eventually defeated the Afghans. The British then redrew the frontier of British India up to the Khyber Pass, and Afghanistan had to yield various frontier areas. The Afghans initiated the fighting in the 3rd Anglo-Afghan war when Amanullah Khan sent troops into British India in 1919. Within a month they had been forced to retreat.

Contrary to popular belief, the Russians did not suffer a major military defeat in Afghanistan. Granted, the Afghan mujahedeen won some important encounters, notably in the Panjshir valley, but they definitely lost others. The truth is that it culminated in a stalemate and neither side decisively defeated the other. The Soviets could have remained in Afghanistan ad infinitum, but they decided to leave when Gorbachev estimated that the war had reached an impasse. Regarding the cost in men, money and international prestige was no longer viable.

The current conflict in Afghanistan began in 2001 in the wake of the catastrophic events of 9/11. The Bush administration's purpose was to eliminate the terrorist threat of al-Qaida's leader, Osama bin Laden. U.S. forces initiated the "War on Terror" by attacking the Taliban on the premise that they were hiding and protecting this wanted terrorist, the evil mastermind behind the attacks on the twin towers. The U.N. Security Council issued punitive sanctions against Afghanistan. These sanctions, along with the ensuing Afghanistan War, may have led to the Taliban's downfall but they were not eliminated. In late December 2014, the NATO combat mission ended and was replaced by an assistance mission baptized "Resolute Support." The name of the mission or operation is largely superfluous to the casualties that are incurred, and with every war there are inevitably casualties; however, improvements in battlefield medicine means that more than 90 percent of soldiers wounded in Afghanistan survive. That's a marked improvement on the Vietnam War's 86.5 percent track record. It is estimated that the cost of veterans' medical and disability payments for the United States alone over the next forty years could reach as high as $1 trillion. Considering that these young men and women are prepared to give everything for the country they served and suffered for, the personal cost to those who return dismembered and disfigured is incalculable.

A war, a conflict, a police action, and an insurgency: all these descriptions are surplus to requirements to the medical teams patching up and reassembling the shattered bodies of young men and women wounded in action. Regardless of the nature or the reason for violent confrontation, they are always required to do their job. In Vietnam nurses and doctors had to deal with injuries that resulted from bullets, bombs, and booby traps. But during the Iraq and Afghan wars, a new menace surfaced that became the cause of a significant percentage of all allied wounded. In the second Iraq War, IEDs (Improvised Explosive Devices) were used extensively against U.S.-led invasion forces and by the end of 2007, they had become responsible for approximately 63 percent of coalition deaths in Iraq.

Between 2001 to the end of 2014, NATO/ISAF coalition forces suffered 1,401 deaths as a result of IEDs, which is around 50.4 percent of their total losses in combat. In the period from 2008 to 2011, IEDs fatalities amounted to between 58 percent and 61 percent of the coalition losses. The number of wounded from IEDs and the casualties among the Afghan forces aren't known but according to data from the Pentagon's Joint IED Defeat Organization (or JIEDDO), between more than half to two-thirds of Americans killed or wounded in combat in the Iraq and Afghanistan wars have been victims of IEDs planted in the ground, in vehicles or buildings, worn as suicide vests, or loaded into suicide vehicles.

The IEDs are assembled using a variety of components that include an initiator, switch, main charge, power source, and a container. IEDs may be surrounded by or packed with additional materials or "enhancements" such as nails, glass, or metal fragments designed to increase the amount of shrapnel propelled by the explosion. Enhancements may also include other elements such as hazardous materials. An IED can be initiated by a variety of methods depending on the intended target. They were originally introduced to Middle East and Central Asia, somewhat paradoxically, by the U.S. military. Iraq insurgents probably learned how to manufacture the deadly devices from the electronically accessible U.S.

Army Technical Manual TM 31-210. They hurriedly improved on the basic American recipes, building a succession of harder to detect, more potent and easier to use contraptions. Iraqi know-how was successfully transferred to Afghanistan and continuously enhanced, both technically and tactically, thus turning IEDs into one of the most effective weapons in the armories of the Taliban. The main issue with IEDs is that it is a weapon that doesn't only hit foreign troops on ground patrols and in road convoys, it's also an indiscriminate terror weapon that kills and maims thousands of civilians.

Treating casualties resulting from contact with IEDs presents new problems for medical teams operating in war zones. Due to its nature and mechanism, an IED has the potential to inflict a multidimensional injury, impairing numerous systems and organs. IED blasts can result in serious permanent or long-lasting disabilities that can result in amputations, internal injuries, burns, brain injury, and psychological trauma. Even though victim activated IEDs have a higher fatality rate than factory made antipersonnel mines, as reported in Afghanistan, they still wound far more people than they kill. Most who survive these explosions will require medical (and in some cases, psychological) assistance for many years to come. Victim-activated IEDs are devices that are detonated by the presence, proximity, or contact of a person or a vehicle.

IEDs are the source of the greatest fear that preoccupies most soldiers entering a war zone. The fear of losing a limb is one thing, but the fear of losing their reproductive organs is greater. The initial blast from an IED has the capacity to sever arms and legs, ripping through soft flesh, crushing organs and bone, and driving dirt, rocks, and filth deep into gaping wounds, it can also mutilate the victims genitals or blow them off completely. Some of 3rd Battalion, 5th Marines guys said they'd rather be dead than suffer that fate.

Knowing that he was earmarked for active duty in Afghanistan, one young, newly-married marine planned to take the precaution of having his sperm frozen so that in the event of contact with an IED, he and his wife would still be able to have children. Sadly, time constraints prevented him from doing this. A few weeks later he was on a combat patrol in Sagging, southern Afghanistan, walking behind an engineer sweeping for IEDs. There was a blinding flash followed by a wave of searing heat. The upward blast ripped off both of the young man's legs and most of his left arm, slashing into his remaining arm, shattering his pelvis, and driving a rock and other debris up into his abdominal cavity. Amid the bloody carnage, all the skin was ripped from his penis and his testicles were gone. Later while recovering in hospital, he called his wife to apologize for the nature of his injuries. Holding back the tears she stoically reassured the wounded soldier and said, "We will pull through this together, as a team."[116]

Despite some of the devastating injuries that occurred to soldiers in the field one particular unit, the British 34 Field Hospital at Camp Bastion claimed a 98 percent survival rate for casualties, making it a world leader in trauma care. Nevertheless, during a standard tour in Afghanistan, there were reports that doctors and nurses, ambulance drivers and paramedics, hospitals and health centers all came under attack at some time or another. This naturally disrupted the delivery of medical care when needed most. Patients (both civilians and combatants) died because they were prevented from receiving necessary care on many occasions.

One of the most disturbing aspects to emerge from recent conflicts is as a result of social media. Soldiers go on patrol wearing head cams that have "live streaming" capabilities, and many carry cell phones. Some of these recordings end up both inadvertently (and purposely) on social media, where many quickly go viral. During the raid on Osama Bin Laden's compound by U.S. Navy Seals, live video footage was allegedly streamed to the White House.

A helmet camera recorded an incident in 2013 that led to the conviction of a British Royal Marine for murder, for the shooting of an unarmed and injured Afghan insurgent. Military authorities regarded the

---

[116] David Wood, "Beyond The Battlefield: Afghanistan's Wounded Struggle With Genital Injuries," HuffPost (Huffington Post, March 21, 2012), https://www.huffpost.com/entry/beyond-the-battlefield-afghanistan-genital-injuries_n_1335356?page=1.

act as being in contravention to the Geneva Convention. The audio/video images were used in evidence at a court martial relating to the incident. Insurgent groups such as so-called Islamic State have been quick to weaponize social media for their own nefarious designs, and these days they use every available platform in a no-holds-barred policy for the purpose of recruitment and disseminating evil propaganda.

CHAPTER NINETEEN

What Lies Beyond?

Battlefield medical experiences procured from the frontline during World War I, World War II, Korea, Vietnam, Iraq, and Afghanistan have all in some way or another influenced what people regard as modern day medicine. In World War I, approximately four of every one hundred wounded men who received treatment could be expected to survive; in World War II that figure rose to fifty of every one hundred. Closer examination of historical casualty rates indicates that almost 50 percent of military personnel that were killed in action died as a result of excessive blood loss. Eighty percent of those succumbed within an hour after initial injury. To a combat medic that first crucial hour is known as the "golden hour." If the surgeon, nurse, or combat medic can treat the hemorrhage within an hour after the initial injury has occurred, the wounded have a far greater chance of survival. For the past two decades, combat medics have trained intensively to keep wounded soldiers alive while bullets and bombs are being exchanged on the reliable assumption that assistance is always just a radio call away, and these days it usually is.

Combat medics still fulfill a bipartisan role when serving on the front lines. They are expected to be trained soldiers and fight alongside their brothers and sisters in arms, but they are also tasked with preserving life on and off the battlefield. They are expected to be both warrior and healer. But it's important to remember that these remarkable individuals are not automatons. They are living, breathing human beings who suffer the same stresses and anxieties as the other soldiers they serve with. They are indeed courageous and tenacious, but they are not invulnerable. Consequently, many suffer from residual post-traumatic stress symptomatology. Despite being revered and considered irrepressible by their peers, they are often deeply affected by their combat experiences. The compulsion to internalize traumatic experiences is heavier among combat medics, but there are inevitably consequences.

Their double-duty role subjects combat medics to stress factors that other military specialties are sometimes oblivious to. The task of continually providing front line aid means that some are at potentially high risk for burnout, compassion fatigue, combat stress, and medic PTSD. The symptoms often rely on "trigger" factors, events, or occasions that cause the sufferer to relive the initial trauma, which can result in feeling on edge, nightmares, or abnormal sleep patterns. These stress reactions are common after a traumatic event and in many cases, they may subside after a couple of months; however, medics with PTSD can experience a whole plethora of related symptoms even years after the event occurs.

This was the case with volunteer Nurse Augusta Chiwy who wasn't a combat medic, just a civilian nurse who inadvertently found herself saving lives on the front line. Seventy years after the events that impacted her life occurred during the Battle of the Bulge, she couldn't even hear the name "Bastogne."

Like other war veterans, many former medics experience depression, anxiety, marital problems, and substance abuse. Those experiencing the effects of PTSD are often inclined to self-medicate with alcohol, prescription medication, or illegal drugs, and in many cases the symptoms don't dissipate with time. Being a combat medic doesn't make one exempt from the dangers of being on the front line; if anything, it exacerbates them. They are not doctors and are perfectly capable of disposing of an enemy combatant when required, which makes them fair game for the opposing forces. If a medic is tending a wounded soldier, it's safe to assume that they are already in a precarious situation and prone to enemy fire.

Despite the fact that throughout the recent decades there have been gargantuan strides made in the advancement of treating chronic and debilitating disease processes, traumatic injuries sustained during active service continue to represent an impracticable balance between basic physiology and time.

Relying on immediate tourniquet utilization, stabilization by "Forward Surgical Teams," and prompt evacuation of wounded to higher levels of care has enabled front line units to increase individual survival rates to a factor of 90 percent, and in some cases when the wounded person was able to make it to a higher level of care, the survival rate was as high as 97 percent.

Talented military commanders always respected the terrain where their armies fought, and the really good ones often used geographical features to their advantage. Prior knowledge of the terrain and environment will inevitably impact how medical services are deployed to support the troops in action because these variable environments will present unique challenges for those providing battlefield first aid.

To deal with emerging weapon technologies, medical care advancements and requirements need to develop concurrently at the same rate. This will inevitably present challenges because diverse terrains will require different approaches. Fighting in an urban environment is significantly different than having to negotiate a mountainous battlefield. Distinguishing the needs for various environments will be a critical element in maintaining future readiness.

Modern medical teams and combat medics are trained to deal with the deleterious effects of repetitive strain injuries and heat exhaustion, and have identified the initial steps in the management of head injuries and urgent limb preservation. Sophisticated algorithms for the care and recovery of the severely injured soldier have advanced throughout the last decade and military medicine continues to innovate.

Maybe the future will see the use and deployment of artificial intelligence in the shape of autonomous systems capable of guiding providers of various skillsets or even directly providing care to the wounded? Modern technology and growth in the understanding of biologic processes, offers tremendous opportunities to combat the scale of and magnitude of battlefield medicine's challenges. A futuristic battle suit with a network that can connect an injured troop with doctors at a hospital potentially thousands of miles away is already being developed. The battle suits are embedded with technology that can track the troop's location, vital signs, and even administer medicine to reduce shock. The information means a Combat Rescue Officer will be able to begin conducting triage even before physically arriving on the scene.

There was a relatively recent case of a healthy twenty-two-year-old male soldier who suffered severe blast injuries to the torso after the nearby detonation of an IED. He was immediately put on a medevac helicopter and placed under the auspices of flight medic for transport to the nearest military surgical hospital, which was roughly fifty kilometers away. Once the wounded soldier was secured inside the helicopter, intravenous drips were applied, and he was given analgesia as the helicopter exited the combat zone under enemy fire. During the wound assessment, the soldier's vital signs registered normal, but after several minutes in transit he began to complain of severe abdominal and chest pain. The flight medic requested more details, but the soldier's utterances were becoming increasingly unintelligible. Moreover, the situation was exacerbated due to the clamorous engine noises of the helicopter.

Within moments the soldier became progressively tachycardic. His oxygen saturation began to deteriorate and his heart rate began to rise. The flight medic performed an e-FAST examination with a portable ultrasound device. The e-FAST examination provided an ability to assess for life-threatening injuries during evacuation. His abdominal and pericardial ultrasonographic windows were negative for the presence of intraperitoneal or pericardial fluid. As the patient's vital signs continued to deteriorate, ultrasound imaging of the thoracic fields revealed the presence of a large right-sided pneumothorax. Right pleural space needle decompression, followed by placement of right-sided tube thoracotomy, placed to suction, was immediately performed, resulting in a normalization of all vital signs. The soldier's life was saved thanks to modern technology.

Despite the introduction of these technologies, contemporary combat medics will still be compelled to prove their efficiency in four major competencies before deploying to the front lines. Emergency care, evacuation, medical force protection, and limited primary care will remain the core knowledge skill of all combat medics. Emergency care implies the accustomed skills of combat casualty care and trauma resuscitation. Specific skills include hemorrhage control, splinting, bandaging, advanced airway management, intravenous fluid therapy, decompression of tension pneumothorax, and shock management.

One US combat medic recently said, "I have had 18 years if service and 3 deployments under me to both Iraq and Afghanistan. The last one in Afghanistan was pretty kinetic. During the first Gulf War I was with a chemical response team in case any chemical weapons were used I was trained as a chemical warfare medic. We were trained to specifically identify chemical agents, their signs and symptoms, and how to decontaminate while still medically treating the casualties. I've noticed over the past 18 years how much the equipment we use has improved but in my opinion it still comes down to training. When I first began training as a medic, to stop bleeding it was always about applying pressure and elevating and in the worst-case scenario you apply a tourniquet. After being at war for a few years our bosses told us to use the tourniquet right away because that saves more lives. The evolution happened very quickly.

"The evolution occurred over four to six years it was a case of, 'Hey look this seems to work better so let's do it.' It's saving more lives on the battlefield so let's do this and train accordingly. So we went from training our guys on the ground, from applying pressure and elevating to hey put the tourniquet on immediately to stop the bleeding because you want to save a life instead of just prevent damage. The triage process became a little more streamlined, a little easier. It's not just the medic that's doing this on the battlefield. The medic is doing the triage, whether it be a medic or a nurse or a doctor or someone who is medically qualified. But you also have other people around who can manage this and they may not be medical personnel but they have the basic training that we call 'Combat lifesaver training' in the US Army, to be able to sustain life. Maybe it's not immediate but then we have something we call a battle buddy who can also apply a tourniquet if there's massive bleeding, and they can apply a chest feel or something like that, and that's kind how it evolved. Sometimes you feel like you're never prepared enough because what we do is so important, we try and take care of casualties the best we can. But unfortunately not all of them can be saved you know, then you always have this feeling of inadequacy, what could I have done better to save this person's life. I never felt when I had a casualty that there was something that I forgot to do or something that I knew how to do that I didn't do. It was always, I wish I would have known how to take care of this person better, or would it have helped or would it have made a difference.

"The way I see I see things evolving is there are a lot of new products that people are coming out with, that after their experiences on the battlefield or experiences themselves. They're coming out with better ways to stop the bleeding because that's the most important, or being able to get them back to a higher echelon of care. The way I see a thing evolving is, way back in the day, back before this war (Afghanistan) started, medics in the military were trained to do all your basic stuff, kinda like what we call I the United States a (inaudible – D&D or T&T basic). They know how to stop bleeding, they know how to give oxygen and they know how to do CPR. It's becoming more advanced now to where they realize the initial point of care when the person was first hit, you know the 'Golden hour' is the most critical. In order to maximize that time, when there is no way you can get someone off the battlefield and into a higher echelon of care. Investing more money and more training into individual. Each individual that is there, and not only investing in the knowledge of the medic that's on the ground but investing in the knowledge of every person around because 9 time out of 10 there's only 1 medic for 20, 35 people. But if everybody knows basic care then they can provide aid until the medic is able to do what they can do.

"As far as advancement is concerned, there may be a few technological advancements, things like that, maybe some new equipment. But I think that the biggest thing that they'll start doing is start investing in the knowledge and the capabilities and allowing the medics on the ground to do more. They already do it with Special Forces Teams and other high efficient teams but they're also going to begin in giving a higher degree of medical knowledge to all the other medics who are on the ground. Being able to transfer that knowledge to everybody else in the platoon is equally important, so that they can help out when they can.

"In my opinion we have gotten better at providing the right kid of treatment at the point of entry and we've been able to enhance the likelihood of survival. This is just my personal opinion based on 18 years of service."[117]

Military planners have long envisaged using robotics on the battlefield, the potential for utilizing parallel technologies suitably developed to enhance the practice of battlefield medicine and trauma care in the future is also in the pipeline. The future may see remote controlled automatons proliferating in ground medical operations where they will have the potential to reduce casualties among combat medics and significantly improve the life-saving effectiveness of medical interventions while in the process further reducing battlefield mortality rates.

As contemporary military planners prepare for contingencies involving operations by sizeable forces for special operations and conflict situations, which may involve a limited military intervention force, the archetypical linear battlefield situation we have known in the past will become antiquated. The potential for new high-tech weaponry, use of chemical and biological agents, along with combatting nontraditional forces and terrorism will demand a totally different approach to deal with what will be perceived as a 360 degree threat.

The general consensus of opinion among the military hierarchy is that the increasing global urbanization of the world's population implies that it's more than likely that future battles will be fought out within city

---

[117] Author interview. Real name withheld for security reasons. Soldier is still on active duty.

limits. Cutting edge advanced technology may indeed pave the way for enhanced combat casualty care, but it will not entirely eliminate the need for human intervention. The combat medics will still carry tourniquets, junctional hemorrhage control devices, and intraosseous needles (used for injecting directly into the marrow of a bone).

Despite all the advances, many of these so-called new tools and concepts have existed in some form or another for centuries, and history should never forget the innovators. Such is the nature of humanity that it's practically inevitable that there will always be wars and conflicts and combatants in harm's way may get wounded. As long as that is the case, the ultimate purpose was, is, and will remain, despite whatever technology is used, the optimization of care on the battlefield. Caring, like courage, can't be programmed into any machine.

CHAPTER TWENTY

Fighting COVID-19

This volume begins in the "New World" and ends in another "New World." No one knows who will prevail and what new world will transpire after the pandemic of 2020. As we have seen in the previous chapters, civilian medical teams and experts have been employed by the U.S. military on numerous occasions. The fight against COVID-19 is no exception; however, the current pandemic isn't the first time U.S. military forces have been requisitioned for domestic emergencies, and there are numerous examples of their use throughout American history. When George Washington urgently dispatched troops to quash an uprising of farmers and distillers protesting a whiskey tax during the Whiskey Rebellion in 1794, he demonstrated that the new federal government had the capacity to suppress and neutralize violent resistance to the implementation of federal laws. It made no odds that those orchestrating the Whiskey Rebellion were justifiably upset (because whiskey is something worth getting very upset about).

Throughout the 19th century, the Army played a pivotal role in enforcing these federal laws and implementing the policies of post–Civil War reconstruction. Most of the uses of the military for domestic purposes have included disaster responses, such as assistance during the devastating Hurricanes Katrina (in 2005) and Sandy (in 2012) and support to the U.S. Forest Service fighting the forest fires in California. The interdepartmental cooperation between civilian and military authorities in the U.S. is still functioning at the highest level.

While the world sits around waiting and hoping for a vaccine or a cure, consideration should be made regarding the nature of this current virus. When it emerged, the virus was known as a "novel" strain of the coronavirus family. Scientists attributed an interim name to the strain of 2019-nCoV, accounting for the year of discovery, its status as a "novel" virus, and its family name (CoV). It's basically a severe mutation of the common cold, for which we have no vaccine. Most people who become ill with the virus will experience mild to moderate symptoms and recover without special treatment, but it can be fatal. Older people and those with preexisting medical conditions (such as high blood pressure, heart problems, or diabetes) appear to be more vulnerable.

The devastating effects of COVID-19 on the health of racial and ethnic minority groups are still emerging, but the most recent data suggests a substantially disproportionate burden of illness and death has been registered among racial and ethnic minority groups. Data accumulated from 580 patients hospitalized with COVID-19 discovered that 45 percent of individuals for whom race or ethnicity data was available were white, compared to 55 percent of individuals in the surrounding community; 33 percent of hospitalized patients were black compared to 18 percent in the community; and 8 percent were Hispanic, compared to 14 percent in the community. These data suggest an overrepresentation of blacks among hospitalized patients. New York City identified death rates among Black/African American persons (92.3 deaths per one hundred thousand population) and Hispanic/Latino persons (74.3) that were substantially higher than that of white (45.2) or Asian (34.5) persons.

One of the explanations given regarding the reasons that racial and ethnic minorities are more vulnerable to the virus is possibly due to the fact that they are more likely to reside in densely populated areas due to institutional racism, which manifests in the form of residential housing segregation. It draws the conclusion that people living in densely pop-ulated areas may find prevention measures such as social distancing difficult to apply and adhere to.

One front line COVID-19 Nurse in New York said, "In all my 38 years as a nurse I never saw anything like this before. I'm worried about those who don't take this seriously. No one is immune but one has to see the effects firsthand to realize how terrible this virus is. Just yesterday I held the hand of a 60-year-old man and watched him struggle to breathe as he slowly lost the fight to hold on to his only life. He squeezed my hand quite tightly seconds before he passed, and I could see, I could actually see how the absolute terror in his eyes reflected the agony of this painful and protracted death. Then he gave me one last look and it was like a strange calm enveloped the room and pain left him. I'm not particularly religious but there's definitely something else at work at such times and I've seen it so often now but every time I have to go through this it tears off a piece of my heart and spits it out.

"We are having a lot of difficulty coping with the' sheers numbers that have been affected. It's really sad when one of our own contracts the virus. I haven't lost anybody close so far but every day I go home worried that I may be carrying the disease. We've lost two so far but there could be more. We're all pulling extra shifts to compensate for the magnitude of admittance due to the coronavirus" [118]

The hospital ship USNS Comfort harbored in New York City. Shortly after arriving from its home port in Norfolk, Virginia, the military's float-ing hospital prepared to receive coronavirus patients. Another hospital ship USNS Mercy (T-AH-19) left Los Angeles seven and a half weeks after arriving at a California epicenter of the COVID-19 pandemic and ten days after discharging its last patient. The medical treatment facility (MTF) staff left sixty-one personnel behind to continue supporting state and local healthcare providers at skilled nursing facilities, at the direction of Federal Emergency Management Agency (FEMA) and U.S. Northern Command (USNORTHCOM). This is one way that civilian and military

---

[118] Author interview: Real name withheld.

authorities and personnel are working together for the same goal to defeat or at least contain and neutralize the same indiscriminate enemy.

The United States military response entailed activating almost forty-seven thousand National Guard soldiers and airmen to fight COVID-19; this pandemic marks the most expansive domestic response to a crisis since Hurricane Katrina. Responding to the pandemic, the National Guard is primarily focused on providing viable COVID-19 testing sites along with the distribution of medical supplies and food. In the month of April 2020, guardsmen packaged, served, or delivered more than forty-four million meals to those in need and transported over thirty-four thousand tons of bulk food to support food banks and other community based programs. At the time of writing the guardsmen have supported 1,600 screening sites nationwide that have tested more than 750,000 people. One medic with a Florida Army National Guard unit said, "As medics, we handle certain challenges that others may not experience. Everyone chose the medical profession for personal reasons, and due to that choice, we are here today helping the citizens of South Florida."[119]

Meanwhile the West Virginia Army National Guard established one of the first Defense Department-approved mobile testing labs. The 20th Chemical, Biological, Radiological, Nuclear, and Explosives Command set to work organizing personal protective equipment for healthcare workers and emergency responders in need. Soldiers joined forces with other volunteers in the Aberdeen Proving Ground, Maryland, to donate their free time and personal 3D printing capabilities to print and create state of the art face shields for give to hospitals and healthcare workers combating COVID-19 across the nation.

When the first wave of people that had symptoms related to COVID-19 turned up at Montefiore Medical Center in the Bronx, one of the managers claimed that he and other nurses had to get by with only two N95 masks per week. This was just one example of the glaring lack of

---

[119] Eric B Smith, "Guard's COVID-19 Response Is Largest since Hurricane Katrina," Washington Headquarters Services, (May 12, 2020), https://www.whs.mil/News/News-Display/Article/2184776/guards-covid-19-response-is-largest-since-hurricane-katrina/.

PPE's in circulation (Personal Protective Equipment). Instead of throwing protective masks away after treating contagious patients, they stored them in paper bags. It's nothing short of staggering that the best funded healthcare system in the world has been sending nurses into wards full to the brim with infected patients without providing basic PPE. There was no excuse; the tardy, lackluster approach of the authorities has actually exacerbated the crisis. The first warning signs emerged in early February 2020, weeks before COVID-19 erupted in the United States. Back then the director general of the WHO (World Health Organization) warned of potentially "severe disruption" in the PPE supply chain due to the demand being one hundred times higher than normal.

Another particularly ominous aspect of the virus is the claim that it targets ethnic minorities. One nurse practitioner was educating seniors on managing their diabetes before he was drawn into the fight against COVID-19 in the heart of New York City. He said, "I have worked during the influenza outbreaks, the swine flu, but never a public health threat of this dimension. April 8 was one of the hardest days"[120] at his hospital, Mount Sinai West. He went on to say that his fluency in Spanish was really useful for dealing with Hispanic patients and their worried families. It is, he says, "very important to offer them information about their loved ones, in a language they can understand. I am tending to a lot of Latino patients with COVID-19."[121]

Preliminary data from city health officials indicates that there are 276,000 Latino nurses are currently working in the United States, which is roughly 10 percent of the health workforce from an ethnic minority that constitutes constitute 18 percent of the population.

This is a global pandemic and different countries around the world have orchestrated different responses. The International Council of Nurses (ICN) claim that at the time of writing, around ninety thousand healthcare workers have been infected by COVID-19 and more than 260 nurses have died due to the pandemic (but they warned that the numbers

---

[120] Kaiser Health News. Twitter Post (April 17, 2020). 12:45 p.m., https://twitter.com/KHNews/status/1251189965675016192.

[121] Idem

could be considerably higher than the figures released by the ICN, which are based on data from thirty countries). It indicates that, on average, 6 percent of all confirmed cases of COVID-19 are among healthcare workers. This is a rough estimate because governments cannot say exactly how many healthcare workers have been affected and that lack of accurate data has led to a serious underestimation of the infection rate among nurses, and the number of deaths incurred as a direct result of the pandemic.

A COVID-19 nurse in New York said, "I've worked as a nurse for almost 10 years, mainly on a hospital's cardiac floor. One day I was assigned to an ad hoc intensive care unit that had previously been used as an observation unit for highly stable patients awaiting test results. Many of the patients in this new Covid-19 unit were on ventilators.

"When I began the shift, a trained intensive care unit nurse was sobbing in the supply closet. She was overwhelmed and appeared extremely anxious, I hadn't worked on her familiar unit in weeks, and had been told that her next shift would be an overnight one. The nurse had no say in the matter. Many of are assigned to work in unfamiliar units, with patients who are suffering from something that is outside our expertise, without any training. We're lost. Most shifts start with nurses crying and most shifts end that way too."[122]

Every day nurses have to deal with the emotionally draining dilemma of informing the family that their loved one has passed or is enduring the final hours of their life. "It's really heartbreaking," said one Californian nurse who went on to say that, "One can only internalize so much heartache so we tend to dissolve into a form of denial. The situation wouldn't be manageable otherwise."

Some notable historians claim that pandemics conclude in one of two ways involving the medical aspect that occurs when the incidence and death rates drop below a certain level and the social aspect when fear of the disease dissipates. The insinuation is that the end of restrictions is not determined by medical and public health data but by sociopolitical processes whereupon people become weary of being constantly in "panic

---

[122] https://www.statnews.com/2020/05/06/nurse-frightened-hospital-administrators-more-than-covid-19/.

mode" and draw their own conclusions as to whether or not it's safe to stop complying with the lockdown and social distancing regulations.

People are, by nature, highly susceptible and vulnerable. The appearance of COVID-19 among global populations has led to a near exponential growth in cases in a very short time. Humanity has survived previous pandemics and will probably learn to deal with this one. All human infectious diseases and pandemics have originated by way of cross species transmission of microorganisms from human to human, animals to humans, and vice versa. It's all fodder for the "doom and Armageddon" mob currently nodding sagely and feeling just a bit vindicated by recent events. Well, one must make hay while the sun shines.

There's another ominous aspect to this virus. The World Health Organization (WHO) said there is "no evidence" that survivors of COVID-19 cannot be re-infected with the virus. In a statement, WHO warned that antibodies may not adequately protect survivors, leaving them vulnerable to a second coronavirus infection. The warning came as several countries, including the United States, are considering allowing people who have recovered to carry "immunity passports" or "risk-free certificates." That documentation would allow survivors to return to work and other activities under the assumption that they are immune from the virus.

A Belgian care worker in a country that actively encourages euthanasia related one of the most worrying and disconcerting aspects of COVID-19. She was afflicted twice by it. She said, "I'm not qualified to give medication. I'm a nursing assistant working in a geriatric care home, but during this pandemic we have been so incredibly busy that I have often been asked by the qualified staff to dose sufferers with powerful sedatives. Some were treated like terminal cancer patients and given extra doses of morphine-based drugs. Like they do here with palliative care. I've seen some terrible things. My colleague explained that the elderly and infirm didn't have much chance of surviving anyway, but it can't be right. I have already had corona but I'm working without sufficient PPE (Personal protective equipment) because I'm infected anyway, I've been infected twice so I get sent to see to all the COVID-19 sufferers. I don't understand. I thought that I was alright but it came back, the disease came back. I feel like shit but I have to work. Thankfully I'm young and I believe that I will survive this God willing, but I will have to live with the sad truth that an old person dying from this terrible disease that consumes their vital organs, is in some cases better off dead. I know that sounds hard but the truth always is."[123]

The U.S. has been one of the worst affected countries of the COVID-19 outbreak in the industrialized world (72.9 percent of those who died with COVID-19 were male, with an average age of 65.8 years and usually afflicted by underlying chronic conditions, such as heart problems or diabetes). The risk groups of males over fifty with chronic comorbid conditions, including hypertension (high blood pressure), coronary heart disease, and diabetes led experts to conclude that every effort must be taken to protect this vulnerable group.

Front line COVID-19 Nurse Allycia King (daughter of author Martin King). Received a letter from former American Ambassador Mrs. Denise Campbell Bauer thanking her for working to save the lives of those injured in the Brussels Airport terrorist attack. Allycia said, "It's bad enough seeing the lives of previously vibrant people ebb away to nothing but we keep stepping up to the plate regardless because it's what we do. We haul and lift patients often much heavier than ourselves. Then there's the abominable PPE (Personal protective equipment) that we are compelled to wear day in day out. It can get very claustrophobic and desperately uncomfortable, a lot of nurses have developed unsightly facial skin rashes due to this equipment. I look forward to the day when all this is over but no doubt there will be other problems to contend with. One can mentally immunize against people dying, it goes with the turf but the immunity isn't permanent and nurses may hide their feelings but trust me they do feel, genuinely feel for the misery and heartache this despicable virus causes. It's dangerous to be complacent or to assume that everything is alright when it isn't, but I have every faith that we will get there.

---

[123] Author interview: Name withheld.

This volume was written during lockdown. This pandemic will end eventually and no doubt there may be fresh challenges ahead. According to history, pandemics traditionally have two types of endings. The first scenario refers to the medical aspect, which occurs when the incidence and death rates plunge, and then the social aspect, when the epidemic of fear about the disease dissipates. At least now the scientific and medical community has a greater capacity to combat disease and vaccines are being rolled out across the world. As long as we have qualified, caring individuals who are willing to step up to the plate when they have to, there is always be hope. There will always be innovations, and they will always be there where and when they are most needed. Bless them all.

ACKNOWLEDGMENTS

Martin King:

First and foremost grateful thanks to my wife Freya, my daughter Nurse Allycia King and my son Ashley, my insiprational agent Roger S. Williams and my long time friends Mike, John and Joanne Collins. Also deep thanks to Kate Monahan, Kiera and the staff at Knox Press for all their invaluable assistance. Thank you also to my respected friends Brigadier General Robert G. Novotny, USAF (ret), Colonel Robert Campbell 101st Airborne (ret) Commander Jeff Barta USN (ret). Veteran Bob Babcock, Karl K. Warner III and the tremendous staff at the U.S. Army Heritage & Education Center for the excellent work they do. Thanks to Peter Snow and Ann MacMillan, Dan Snow, Margaret MacMillan and Sir Max Hastings for keeping history alive and for all the kind words.. Warm thanks to Brian G. Dick the Ambassador and staff at Protocol US Embassy Brussels.

Thank you also to my beloved family and friends in no order of preference, Sandra King and Mick, Rachel Denny, Debbie, Marc, Ben, Becky and Pippa Drury, Graham King and Ann Lawson, Andy and Joe Kirton, George Lee, Alex Ramael, Dirk de Groof and family.Not forgetting fellow authors Charles Harris and Rick Beyer. Excellent history teachers John Taylor, Martina Steffens Taylor and the amazing SHAPE

Middle school kids. Meg Porter and Lori Urbanek for inviting me to their schools. Gone but not forgotten, Mark William Altmeyer and beloved friend 106th Inf Div veteran John R Shaffner and Medal of Honor recipient Francis S. Currey.30th Inf. Div.

Finally a big thank you to the all those excellent doctors and nurses who kept me alive despite the odds. God bless all doctors and nurses.

Michael Collins:

Thank You to my awesome son, Daniel who continues to show me why history is important to pass on to future generations. To my co-author Martin for your support, patience, and as always friendship. My agent Roger Williams for your help during the publication of this book. Our managing editor Kate Monahan for your guidance throughout the editing and publication process. Thank you to my parents John and Joanne Collins, brothers John and Chris, sisters-in-law Melissa and Maria, nieces Morgan, Katie, Keira, and Margo, nephew Henry, and my aunt Pat for your support during the writing of this book. Thanks to all my friends and family who have provided help both here and abroad. Thank you to my father Dr. John A. Collins III, my late grandmother Helen Collins, my cousin Maureen Bridgman, and all the medical personnel in my family for taking care of those in need. In loving memory of my godmother Mary McDonagh and her son Jeffrey McDonagh.